DIABETIC AIR FRYER COOKBOOK

150 EASY AND HEALTHY AIR FRYER RECIPES FOR PEOPLE WITH DIABETES, PLUS A 30-DAYS MEAL PLAN

VANESSA JENSEN

Table of Contents

Introduction

Diabetes is a disease with many names, but for this book's purposes, the term diabetes will mean diabetes mellitus. The word diabetes means "sugar," which refers to a disease characterized by high blood sugar. Diabetes is usually diagnosed by finding out that a patient's blood sugar is higher than normal. There are two main types of diabetes — type 1 and type 2. Type 1 diabetes is an autoimmune disease, so your body's immune system turns on itself. In this form of diabetes, your body stops making insulin, a hormone that helps your body absorb the sugar in food to produce energy. Type 1 is lifelong and always requires treatment.

Type 2 diabetes is an illness where either no longer has enough insulin or can't use it effectively. A primary cause of type 2, which can also affect adults and children, is obesity, which affects the body to lose its ability to use insulin properly. If you have type 2 diabetes, you must take proper care of yourself to prevent complications such as damage to the eyes, heart, blood vessels, or kidney failure. Diabetes control can prevent these complications.

The Diabetes Air Fryer Cookbook was written as a guide for those who are new to the world of air fryers and want to learn what they can do with them. It takes information from a variety of sites and eBooks. We hope you find this book helpful in understanding your new air fryer and how you can make great meals in it!

Are you a diabetic who loves to cook? If so, you know that you have to take special care when preparing your meals. But your diabetic air fryer can make cooking easier and healthier for you. This is because your diabetic air fryer can cook your food without oil or grease. This is great for people on a low-fat diet or just trying to eat less fat-laden foods. But it also makes using your air fryer easier and safer for those with diabetes.

The number of options and benefits offered by your diabetic air fryer is astounding. With this device, you can cook a wide range of foods that previously may have been forbidden because of high fat or sugar levels. With an air fryer, you can prepare ready-to-eat meals that are healthy and nutritious for you. They also take less time to prepare than traditional oven or stovetop cooking methods, making them perfect for busy people like students, commuters, and shift workers.

The benefits extend beyond healthier food, though — they can help you lose weight and cut down on your "bad" cholesterol and triglycerides levels! This makes using your air fryer both healthier and more cost-effective than other cooking methods.

Chapter 1.   What is Diabetes?

Diabetes is a well-being condition that occurs when the body's blood glucose is high. Glucose is a source of energy for your body. Think of your body as a car that needs gasoline as fuel to help it move. Insulin, a hormone made in the pancreas, transports glucose from the bloodstream to the cells where it will be used as energy.

When your body doesn't make enough insulin, doesn't make insulin, or can't use the insulin made the proper way, you will develop diabetes. This will cause a buildup in the blood, stopping glucose from getting into cells for energy.

Types of Diabetes

Type 1 Diabetes

A deficiency of the immune system results in Type 1 diabetes, also called insulin-dependent diabetes or juvenile diabetes. In the pancreas, your immune system destroys the insulin-producing cells, killing the body's capacity to create insulin. It's not clear what causes autoimmune disease and how to treat it effectively. Take insulin to survive with Type 1 diabetes. As an infant or young adult, several individuals are diagnosed. The body shows on the onset of type 1 diabetes are polyuria (excessive excretion of urine), polydipsia (extreme thirst), sudden weight loss, and constant hunger, fatigue, and vision changes. These changes can occur suddenly.

Type 2 Diabetes

Type 2 diabetes, formerly denoted as adult-onset diabetes or non-insulin-dependent, stems from insufficient insulin utilization by the body. Type 2 diabetes is found in most individuals with diabetes. The symptoms can be identical to those with type 1 diabetes. However, much less marked, as a result, the condition can be detected after many years of diagnosis when symptoms have already occurred.

Type 2 diabetes happens when sugar adds up in your blood, and the body becomes resistant to insulin. Type 2 diabetes is insulin resistance, which ultimately leads to obesity; obesity is a collection of different diseases. Older generations were more susceptible, but more and younger generations are now being affected. This is a product of poor health, not enough nutrition, and fitness patterns. Your pancreas avoids using insulin properly in type 2 diabetes. This creates complications with sugar that has to be taken out of the blood and placing it for energy in the cells. Finally, this will add to the need for insulin treatment.

Earlier stages, such as prediabetic, can be controlled successfully through food, exercise, and dynamic blood sugar control. This will also avoid the overall progression of type 2 diabetes. It is possible to monitor diabetes. If sufficient adjustments to the diet are created, the body will receive remission.

Gestational Diabetes

Hyperglycemia with blood glucose levels over average, but below those diabetes levels is diagnosed with gestational diabetes. Gestational diabetes is identified via prenatal tests rather than by signs recorded — high blood sugar, which also occurs during gestation. Hormones produced by the placenta are insulin-blocking, which is the major cause of this type of diabetes. You can manage gestational diabetes most of the time by food and exercise. Usually, it gets resolved after delivery. During pregnancy, gestational diabetes will raise the risk of complications. It will also increase the likelihood that both mothers and infants may experience type 2 diabetes later in life. Insulin-blocking hormones shaped by the placenta cause this type of diabetes.

Causes of Diabetes

Your cells can become immune to insulin's effect in prediabetic, which can happen in type 2 diabetes, and the pancreas cannot generate sufficient insulin to counteract this resistance. Sugar constructs up in your bloodstream instead of going to your cells, where it's required for fuel. It is unclear why this arises, while hereditary and environmental influences are thought to play a role in the progress of type 2 diabetes. The advancement of type 2 diabetes is closely related to being overweight, although not everybody with type 2 is obese. Several variables, including dietary conditions and genetic makeup, handle the most prevalent type of diabetes.

Here are a few factors:

Insulin Resistance

Type 2 diabetes commonly progresses with insulin resistance, a disease in which insulin is not handled well by the body, liver, and fat cells. To enable glucose to reach cells, the body requires more insulin. The pancreas initially generates more insulin to maintain the additional demand. The pancreas cannot create enough insulin over time, and blood glucose levels increase.

Overweight, Physical Inactivity, and Obesity

When you are not regularly involved and are obese or overweight, you are much more prone to have type 2 diabetes. Often, excess weight induces insulin resistance, prominent in persons with type 2 diabetes. In which area of the body stores fat counts a lot. Insulin tolerance, type 2 diabetes, and heart and blood artery dysfunction are attributed to excess belly fat.

Genes and Family History

A family history of diabetes in the family makes it more probable that gestational diabetes may occur in a mother, which means that genes play a part. In African Americans, Asians, American Indians, and Latinas, Hispanic, mutations can also justify why the disease happens more frequently.

Any genes can make you more susceptible to advance type 2 diabetes to type 1 diabetes.

Genetic makeup can make a person more obese, which in turn leads to having type 2 diabetes.

Signs of Having a Diabetes

Many of the same unmistakable warning signals are present with all forms of diabetes.

Itchy skin and Dry mouth: Since the body requires water to urinate, most items provide less moisture. You can get dehydrated, and that might make your mouth taste dry. And dehydration also makes skin dry, which makes you itchy.

Tiredness and Hunger: Your body transforms the food you consume into (sugar) glucose that body cells use for fuel. But insulin is required by your cells to take in glucose. And if the body does not produce enough or none of the insulin or the insulin body produces is immune to your cells, the glucose can't get into them, and you don't have energy. This will leave you hungrier than normal and more drained.

Urinating and Getting Thirstier: Peeing and getting thirstier most frequently. Typically, the average person needs to pee 4 to 7 times in one day, although developing diabetes may go a lot faster because normally, when it moves into your liver, your body reabsorbs glucose. But as diabetes drives your blood sugar up, it may not be practical for your kidneys to get it all backdown. This allows more urine to be created by the liver, and it requires fluids. The outcome: you're going to have to urinate more frequently. You will get thirsty when you urinate too much. Hence drinking more water.

Blurred Vision: As your body cannot process fluids more efficiently, which leads to the swelling of lenses in your eyes. Hence, they have changed shape and cannot focus as before. It results in blurred vision.

Hence, to prevent the onset of diabetes, it is important to eat healthily, stay active, eat less junk food, and monitor your blood glucose levels regularly.

Obesity and Diabetes

Diabetes is a stubborn condition that arises from 2 reasons: when the pancreas cannot produce insulin enough for body needs or whenever the body's insulin may not be used properly. Insulin is a blood sugar-regulating hormone. Hyperglycemia, or high blood sugar, is a typical result of uncontrolled diabetes, causing significant harm to the body's structures, especially blood vessels and nerves. Diabetes mellitus is a category of illness that influences how the body uses glucose. Glucose is essential to your well-being. The cells that create up the muscles and tissues require a significant glucose supply. It's the brain's primary power supply, too. The primary issue of diabetes varies based on the type of diabetes. And this can cause excessive sugar in the blood, no matter what diabetes a person has. If there is too much sugar, it can lead to grave health issues. The insulin hormone transfers the sugar into the cells from the blood.

High blood sugar levels may cause harm to your kidneys, eyes, organs, and nerves.

To understand the major reason for diabetes, know the body's normal glucose consumption route.

How to Prevent?

Type 1 Diabetes cannot currently be prevented; no preventive strategy has proven effective. However, preventive action for conditions like Type 2 Diabetes which are believed to help prevent Type 1 Diabetes includes these:

- Prefer foods low in fat and calories; consume fruit and vegetables in abundance.
- Engage in moderate aerobic physical activity for at least 20 to 30 minutes per day (or 150 minutes per week).
- I was keeping fit weight, avoiding conditions like overweight and obesity.

Chapter 2.   What Is Air Frying?

An air fryer is comparable to an oven in how it roasts and bakes. Still, the distinction is that the heating elements are situated only on top and supported by a strong, large fan, which results in very crisp food in no time. The air fryer uses spinning-heated air to easily and uniformly cook food instead of using a pot of hot oil. To encourage the hot air to flow evenly around the meal, the meal is put in a metal basket (mesh) or a rack, producing the same light golden, crispy crunch you get from frying in oil. It is easy to use air fryers. Besides, they cook food faster than frying and clean up quickly. You can prepare a selection of healthy foods such as fruits, beef, seafood, poultry, and more, besides making beneficial variants of your favorite fried foods such as chips, onion rings, or French fries.

The air fryer is the modern kitchen tool that is proving its worth in effectively reducing the risk of diabetes, weight loss, and living a healthier life without compromising on fried, fatty, and high-calorie food.

How it Works

The air fryer is a convective heat oven with a revved-up countertop. Its small room enables cooking much quicker. A heating device and a fan are kept at the top of the device. Hot air flows through and around food put in a basket-type fryer. This fast circulation, just like deep frying, renders the food crisp. It's also super quick to clean up, and most systems include dishwasher-safe components.

Tips for Cooking

Shake the Basket: open the fryer and move food around while cooking in the device's tray, squeezing smaller foods such as French fries and chips. Toss them every 5–10 minutes for better performance.

Do not overcrowd the Basket: Giving plenty of room to foods so that the air will efficiently circulate is what gets you crispy outcomes.

Spray oil on the Food: Make sure the food doesn't cling to the bowl; gently brush foods with cooking spray.

Keep the Food Dry: To prevent splattering and excessive smoke, make sure food is dry before frying (even if you marinate it). In the same way, be sure to remove the grease from the bottom of the machine regularly while preparing high-fat items such as chicken wings.

Know Other Functions of Air Frying: The air fryer is not just for frying, it is also perfect for other healthier cooking methods, such as grilling, baking, and roasting.

Few other tips are:

- Cut the food into equally sized parts for uniform cooking.
- Distribute the food in one thin, even layer in the air fryer basket. If crowded the basket, food can be less crispy.
- A tiny amount of oil would create the same light, golden, crispy crust from frying. I use cooking spray or an oil mister to apply a thin, even coating oil to the food.
- The air fryer is useful for reheating foods, particularly with a crispy crust that you want.

Benefits of Air Fryer with Diabetes

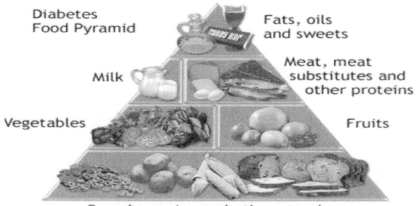

According to this food pyramid, you must consume a large portion of healthy vegetables and whole-grain starches, a balanced amount of healthy fats, and proteins with small amounts of nuts and oils.

Benefits:
- Easy cleanup
- Low-fat meals
- Less oil is needed
- Hot air cooks food evenly
- Weight loss
- Reduced cancer risk
- Diabetes management
- Improved memory
- Improved gut health

Chapter 3.   Breakfast Recipes

1.   Hard-Boiled Eggs

Preparation Time: 2 minutes
Cooking Time: 10 minutes
Servings: 6 eggs

Ingredients:
- 6 pieces eggs

Directions:
1. Arrange raw eggs on the rack of your air fryer, giving at least enough space to circulate the surrounding air.
2. Cook the eggs for fifteen minutes in the fryer at 260°F.
3. Remove the boiled eggs from the fryer and submerge them in a bowl with an ice-water bath for 10 minutes. Peel the eggs and serve.
4. Enjoy!

Nutrition:
- Calories: 62
- Fat: 4 g (1 g saturated fat)
- Cholesterol: 163 mg
- Sodium: 62 mg
- Protein: 5 g.

2.   Grilled Cheese Sandwiches

Preparation Time: 2 minutes
Cooking Time: 10 minutes
Servings: 2 sandwiches

Ingredients:
- 4 slices American cheese
- 4 slices sandwich bread
- Pat Butter

Directions:
1. Warm your air fryer to 360°F.
2. Fill the center of 2 bread slices with two slices of American cheese.
3. Binge an even layer of butter on each side of the sandwich and position it in the hamper of your air fryer in a single layer.
4. Insert toothpicks on the corners of each sandwich to seal.
5. Air-fries the sandwiches for 4 minutes, flipping once, and cook for another 3 to 4 minutes until toasted.
6. Serve!

Nutrition:
- Calories: 297
- Fat: 14.6 g (7.5 g saturated fat)
- Cholesterol: 39 mg
- Sodium: 832 mg
- Carbohydrates: 31.3 g
- Dietary Fiber: 1 g
- Total sugars: 7.1 g
- Protein: 11.8 g.

3.   Hot Dogs

Preparation Time: 2 minutes
Cooking Time: 10 minutes
Servings: 4

Ingredients:
- 4 beef hot dogs

Directions:
1. Using a knife, score the hot dogs to create several little slits to prevent bursting during cooking.
2. Lay the hotdogs in the air fryer.
3. Bake for 5 minutes at 375°F.
4. When the timer is up, rotate the hotdogs; cook for 3 minutes longer.
5. Remove from fryer and dig in.
6. Serve!

Nutrition:
- Calories: 111
- Fat: 6 g (2 g saturated fat)
- Cholesterol: 20 mg
- Sodium: 307 mg
- Carbohydrates: 8 g
- Protein: 4 g.

4.   Perfect Cinnamon Toast

Preparation Time: 2 minutes
Cooking Time: 10 minutes
Servings: 6 slices

Ingredients:
- 1 butter stick, room temperature
- 1 ½ tsp pure vanilla extract
- 1 ½ tsp ground cinnamon
- ½ cup white sugar
- 1 tiny pinch kosher salt
- 2 pinches freshly ground black pepper
- 12 slices whole-wheat bread

Directions:
1. Using the back of your spoon, mash the butter until softened.
2. Add the sugar, vanilla, salt, cinnamon and optional pepper, and stir to combine fully.

3. Spread about 1/6 of the butter mixture onto the bread, covering up to the edges.
4. Load the bread slices into the air fryer basket and cook for 5 minutes at 400°F.
5. Remove toasted bread from the fryer.
6. Cut diagonally and serve while hot.
7. Enjoy!

Nutrition:
- Calories: 355
- Fat: 17 g (10 g saturated fat)
- Cholesterol: 40 mg
- Sodium: 432 mg
- Carbohydrates: 45 g
- Dietary Fiber: 3 g
- Total Sugars: 20 g
- Protein: 6 g.

5. Monkey Bread

Preparation Time: 2 minutes
Cooking Time: 10 minutes
Servings: 8
Ingredients:
- 1 cup non-fat Greek yogurt
- 1 cup self-rising flour
- 1 tsp sugar
- ½ tsp cinnamon

Directions:
1. Combine in a medium bowl the self-rising flour and yogurt; mix well to form into dough.
2. Custom the dough into a large ball and cut into fourths.
3. Remove each dough wedge to shape into a flattened circular disc, and then cut into eight pieces, similar to a pizza. Remove each wedge from the disc and roll it to form into balls.
4. Combine cinnamon and sugar in a Ziploc or resealable plastic bag. Add the dough balls and seal the bag; shake to coat the balls well.
5. Prepare a mini loaf pan by lightly misting it with non-stick spray.
6. Arrange the dough balls in the pan and sprinkle lightly with the sugar-cinnamon mix.
7. Put the loaf pan inside the air fryer. Bake the bread for 7 minutes, at 375°F. Let cool.
8. Enjoy!

Nutrition:
- Calorie: 73
- Sodium: 6 mg
- Carbohydrates: 14.4 g
- Dietary Fiber: 0.5 g
- Total Sugars: 2.4 g
- Protein: 3.1 g.

6. Air Fryer Bacon

Preparation Time: 2 minutes
Cooking Time: 10 minutes
Servings: 5
Ingredients:
- 5 slices (thick-cut) bacon

Directions:
1. Lay the bacon slices into your air fryer basket, at least 1 inch apart, to cook.
2. Heat the air fryer at 390°F.
3. Cook the bacon for 10 to 12 minutes until crispy.
4. Drain on a kitchen napkin before serving.
5. Enjoy!

Nutrition:
- Calories: 103
- Fat: g (2.6 g saturated fat)
- Cholesterol: 21 mg
- Sodium: 439 mg
- Carbohydrate: 0.3 g
- Dietary Fiber: 0 g
- Total Sugars: 0 g
- Protein: 7 g.

7. Meatballs in Tomato Sauce

Preparation Time: 10 minutes
Cooking Time: 10 minutes
Servings: 3–4
Ingredients:
- 1 egg
- ¾ lb. lean ground beef
- 1 onion, chopped
- 3 Tbsp breadcrumbs
- ½ Tbsp fresh thyme leaves, chopped
- ½ cup tomato sauce
- 1 Tbsp parsley, chopped
- Pinch salt
- Pinch pepper, to taste

Directions:
1. Preheat the Air Fryer to 390°F
2. Place all ingredients in a bowl. Mix until well-combined. Divide mixture into 12 balls. Place them in the cooking basket.
3. Cook meatballs for 8 minutes.
4. Put the cooked meatballs in an oven dish. Pour the tomato sauce on top. Put the oven dish inside the cooking basket of the Air Fryer.
5. Cook for 5 minutes at 330°F.

Nutrition:
- Calorie: 129
- Carbohydrate: 15.4 g

- Fat: 17.8 g
- Protein: 17.6 g
- Fiber: 1.2 g

8. Chicken Fried Spring Rolls

Preparation Time: 20 minutes
Cooking Time: 10 minutes
Servings: 4

Ingredients:
For the spring roll wrappers:
- 1 egg, beaten
- 8 spring roll wrappers
- 1 tsp cornstarch
- ½ tsp olive oil

For the filling:
- 1 cup chicken breast, cooked, shredded
- 1 celery stalk, sliced thinly
- 1 carrot, sliced thinly
- 1 tsp chicken stock powder, low sodium
- ½ tsp ginger, chopped finely
- ½ cup sliced mushrooms

Directions:
1. Preheat the Air Fryer to 390°F.
2. Prepare the filling. In a bowl, combine shredded chicken, mushrooms, carrot and celery. Add in chicken, stock powder and ginger. Stir well.
3. Meanwhile, mix cornstarch and egg until thick in a bowl. Set aside.
4. Spoon some filling into a spring roll wrapper. Roll and seal the ends with the egg mixture.
5. Light brush spring rolls with oil and place them in the cooking basket.
6. Cook for 4 minutes. Serve.

Nutrition:
- Calorie: 150
- Carbohydrate: 18 g
- Fat: 5 g
- Protein: 9 g
- Fiber: 1.5 g

9. Mushroom and Cheese Frittata

Preparation Time: 20 minutes
Cooking Time: 10 minutes
Servings: 4

Ingredients:
- 6 eggs
- 6 cups button mushrooms, sliced thinly
- 1 red onion, sliced into thin rounds
- 6 Tbsp Feta cheese, reduced fat, crumbled
- Pinch salt

- 2 Tbsp Olive oil

Directions:
1. Preheat Air Fryer to 330°F.
2. Sauté onions and mushrooms. Transfer to a plate with a paper towel.
3. Meanwhile, beat the eggs in a bowl.
4. Season with salt. Coat a baking dish with cooking spray. Pour egg mixture.
5. Add in mushrooms and onions. Top with crumbled feta cheese.
6. Place baking dish in the Air fryer basket. Cook for 20 minutes. Serve.

Nutrition:
- Calorie: 140
- Carbohydrate: 5.4 g
- Fat: 10.6 g
- Protein: 22.7 g
- Fiber: 1.2 g

10. Cinnamon and Cheese Pancake

Preparation Time: 5–7 minutes
Cooking Time: 10 minutes
Servings: 4

Ingredients:
- 2 eggs
- 2 cups cream cheese, reduced-fat
- ½ tsp cinnamon
- 1 pack Stevia

Directions:
1. Preheat Air Fryer to 330°F.
2. Meanwhile, combine cream cheese, cinnamon, eggs, and stevia in a blender.
3. Pour ¼ of the mixture in the air fryer basket. Cook for 2 minutes on each side. Repeat the process with the rest of the mix. Serve.

Nutrition:
- Calorie: 140
- Carbohydrate: 5.4 g
- Fat: 10.6 g
- Protein: 22.7 g
- Fiber: 1.2 g

11. Low-Carl White Egg and Spinach Frittata

Preparation Time: 12-15 minutes
Cooking Time: 10 minutes
Servings: 4

Ingredients:
- 8 egg whites
- 2 cups fresh spinach
- 2 Tbsp olive oil

- 1 green pepper, chopped
- 1 red pepper, chopped
- ½ cup feta cheese, reduced fat, crumbled
- ¼ yellow onion, chopped
- 1 tsp salt
- 1 tsp pepper

Directions:
1. Warm the Air Fryer to 330°F.
2. Meanwhile, place red and green peppers and onions in the Air Fryer basket, and cook for 3 minutes. Season with salt and pepper.
3. Pour egg whites and cook for 4 minutes. Add in the spinach and feta cheese on top.
4. Cook for 5 minutes.
5. Transfer to a plate, slice, and service.

Nutrition:
- Calorie: 120
- Carbohydrate: 13 g
- Fat: 4.5 g
- Protein: 9.9 g
- Fiber: 1.2 g

12. Scallion Sandwich

Preparation Time: 10 minutes
Cooking Time: 10 minutes
Servings: 1
Ingredients:
- 2 slices wheat bread
- 2 tsp butter, low fat
- 2 scallions, sliced thinly
- 1 Tbsp parmesan cheese, grated
- 3/4 cup cheddar cheese, reduced-fat, grated

Directions:
1. Preheat the Air fryer to 356°F.
2. Spread butter on a slice of bread. Place inside the cooking basket with the butter side facing down.
3. Place cheese and scallions on top. Spread the rest of the butter on the other slice of bread, put it on top of the sandwich, and sprinkle with parmesan cheese.
4. Cook for 10 minutes.

Nutrition:
- Calorie: 154
- Carbohydrate: 9 g
- Fat: 2.5 g
- Protein: 8.6 g
- Fiber: 2.4 g

13. Lean Lamb and Turkey Meatballs with Yogurt

Preparation Time: 10 minutes
Cooking Time: 10 minutes
Servings: 4
Ingredients:
- 1 egg white
- 4 oz. ground lean turkey
- 1 lb. of lean ground lamb
- 1 tsp both cayenne pepper, ground coriander, red chili pastes, salt, and ground cumin
- 2 garlic cloves, minced
- 1 ½ Tbsp parsley, chopped
- 1 Tbsp mint, chopped
- ¼ cup of olive oil

For the yogurt:
- 2 Tbsp of buttermilk
- 1 garlic clove, minced
- ¼ cup mint, chopped
- ½ cup Greek yogurt, non-fat
- Salt, to taste

Directions:
1. Set the Air Fryer to 390°F.
2. Blend all the ingredients for the meatballs in a bowl. Roll and mound them into golf-size round pieces. Arrange in the cooking basket.
3. Cook for 8 minutes.
4. While waiting, combine all the ingredients for the mint yogurt in a bowl. Mix well.
5. Serve the meatballs with mint yogurt. Top with olives and fresh mint.

Nutrition:
- Calorie: 154
- Carbohydrate: 9 g
- Fat: 2.5 g
- Protein: 8.6 g
- Fiber: 2.4 g

14. Air Fried Eggs

Preparation Time: 15 minutes
Cooking Time: 10 minutes
Servings: 4
Ingredients:
- 4 eggs
- 2 cups baby spinach, rinsed
- 1 Tbsp extra-virgin olive oil
- ½ cup cheddar cheese, reduced-fat, shredded, divided
- Bacon, sliced
- Pinch salt

- Pinch pepper

Directions:
1. Preheat the Air Fryer to 350°F.
2. Warm oil in a pan over medium-high flame. Cook the spinach until wilted. Drain the excess liquid. Put the cooked spinach into four greased ramekins.
3. Add a slice of bacon to each ramekin, crack an egg, and put cheese on top.
4. Season with salt and pepper.
5. Put the ramekins inside the cooking basket of the Air Fryer.
6. Cook for 15 minutes.

Nutrition: facts:
- Calorie: 106
- Carbohydrate: 10 g
- Fat: 3.2 g
- Protein: 9.0 g
- Fiber: 1.2 g

15. Cinnamon Pancake

Preparation Time: 15 minutes
Cooking Time: 10 minutes
Servings: 4

Ingredients:
- 2 eggs
- 2 cups cream cheese, reduced-fat
- ½ tsp cinnamon
- 1 pack Stevia

Directions:
1. Preheat Air Fryer to 330°F.
2. Combine cream cheese, cinnamon, eggs and stevia in a blender.
3. Pour ¼ of the mixture in the air fryer basket.
4. Cook for 2 minutes on each side.
5. Repeat the process with the rest of the mixture. Serve.

Nutrition:
- Calorie: 106
- Carbohydrate: 10 g
- Fat: 3.2 g
- Protein: 9.0 g
- Fiber: 1.2 g

16. Spinach and Mushrooms Omelet

Preparation Time: 15 minutes
Cooking Time: 10 minutes
Servings: 4

Ingredients:
- ½ cup spinach leaves
- 1 cup mushrooms
- 3 green onions
- 1 cup water
- ½ tsp turmeric
- ½ red bell pepper
- 2 Tbsp butter, low fat
- 1 cup of almond flour
- ½ tsp onion powder
- ½ tsp garlic powder
- ½ tsp fresh ground black pepper
- ¼ tsp ground thyme
- 2 Tbsp extra-virgin olive oil
- 1 tsp black salt
- Salsa, store-bought

Directions:
1. Preheat the Air Fryer to 300°F.
2. Rinse spinach leaves over tap water. Set aside.
3. In a mixing bowl, combine green onions, onion powder, garlic powder, red bell pepper, mushrooms, turmeric, thyme, olive oil, salt, and pepper. Mix well.
4. In another bowl, combine water and flour to form a smooth paste.
5. In a pan, heat olive oil. Sauté peppers and mushrooms for 3 minutes. Tip in spinach and cook for 3 minutes. Set aside.
6. Put in the air fryer basket our Omelette batter. Cook for 3 minutes before flipping. Place vegetables on top. Season with salt. Serve with salsa on the side.

Nutrition:
- Calorie: 110
- Carbohydrate: 9 g
- Fat: 1.3 g
- Protein: 5.4 g
- Fiber: 1.0 g

17. All Berries Pancakes

Preparation Time: 15 minutes
Cooking Time: 10 minutes
Servings: 4

Ingredients:
- ½ cup frozen blueberries, thawed
- ½ cup frozen cranberries, thawed
- 1 cup coconut milk
- 2 Tbsp coconut oil, for greasing
- 2 Tbsp stevia
- 1 cup whole wheat flour, finely milled
- 1 Tbsp baking powder
- 1 tsp vanilla extract
- ¼ tsp salt

Directions:
1. Preheat Air Fryer to 330°F.
2. In a mixing bowl, combine coconut oil, coconut milk, flour, stevia, baking powder, vanilla extract, and salt. Gently fold in berries.
3. Divide batter into equal portions. Pour into the Air fryer basket. Flip once the edges are set. Do not press down on pancakes.
4. Transfer to a plate. Sprinkle with palm sugar. Serve.

Nutrition:
- Calorie: 57
- Carbohydrate: 14 g
- Fat: 0.3 g
- Protein: 0.7 g
- Fiber: 2.4 g

18.   Cinnamon Overnight Oats

Preparation Time: 5 minutes, plus overnight to refrigerate
Cooking Time: 0 minutes
Servings: 2

Ingredients:
- 2/3 cup unsweetened almond milk
- 2/3 cup rolled oats
- ½ apple, cored and finely chopped
- 2 Tbsp chopped walnuts
- 1 tsp cinnamon
- Pinch sea salt

Directions:
1. In a single-serving container or Mason jar, combine all the ingredients and mix well.
2. Cover and refrigerate overnight.

Nutrition:
- Calories: 242
- Total Fat: 12 g
- Saturated Fat: 1 g
- Sodium: 97 mg
- Carbohydrates: 30 g
- Fiber: 6 g
- Protein: 6 g

19.   Ham and Cheese English muffin Melt

Preparation Time: 10 minutes
Cooking Time: 5 minutes
Servings: 2

Ingredients:
- 1 whole-grain English muffin, split and toasted
- 2 tsp Dijon mustard
- 2 slices tomato
- 4 thin slices deli ham
- ½ cup shredded Cheddar cheese
- 2 large eggs, fried (optional)

Directions:
1. Preheat the oven broiler on high.
2. Spread each toasted English muffin half with 1 tsp of mustard and place them on a rimmed baking sheet, cut-side up.
3. Top each with a tomato slice and 2 slices of ham. Sprinkle each with half of the cheese.
4. Broil in the warmed oven until the cheese melts, 2 to 3 minutes.
5. Serve immediately, topped with a fried egg, if desired.

Nutrition:
- Calories: 234
- Total Fat: 13 g
- Saturated Fat: 7 g
- Sodium: 834 mg
- Carbohydrates: 16 g
- Fiber: 3 g
- Protein: 16 g

20.   Asparagus Omelet

Preparation Time: 10 minutes
Cooking Time: 8 minutes
Servings: 2

Ingredients:
- 3 eggs
- 5 steamed asparagus tips
- 2 Tbsp of warm milk
- 1 Tbsp parmesan cheese, grated
- Salt and pepper, to taste
- Non-stick cooking spray

Directions:
1. Mix in a large bowl, eggs, cheese, milk, salt, and pepper, then blend them.
2. Spray a baking pan with non-stick cooking spray.
3. Transfer the egg mixture into the pan and add the asparagus, then place the pan inside the baking basket.
4. Set the air fryer to 320°F for 8 minutes.
5. Serve warm.

Nutrition:
- Calories: 231
- Total Fat: 9.2 g
- Carbs: 8 g
- Protein: 12.2 g

21.   Pumpkin Pie French toast

Preparation Time: 10 minutes
Cooking Time: 20 minutes
Servings: 4
Ingredients:

- 2 larges, beaten eggs
- 4 slices cinnamon swirl bread
- ¼ cup milk
- ¼ cup pumpkin puree
- ¼ tsp pumpkin spices
- ¼ cup butter

Directions:

1. In a large mixing bowl, mix milk, eggs, pumpkin puree, and pie spice.
2. Whisk until the mixture is smooth. In the egg mixture, dip the bread on both sides.
3. Place the rack inside of the air fryer's cooking basket.
4. Place 2 slices of bread onto the rack. Set the temperature to 340°F for 10 minutes.
5. Serve pumpkin pie toast with butter.

Nutrition:

- Calories: 212
- Total Fat: 8.2 g
- Carbs: 7 g
- Protein: 11.3 g

22.   Breakfast Cheese Bread Cups

Preparation Time: 10 minutes
Cooking Time: 15 minutes
Servings: 2
Ingredients:

- 2 eggs
- 2 Tbsp cheddar cheese, grated
- Salt and pepper, to taste
- 1 ham slice, cut into 2 pieces
- 4 bread slices, flatten with a rolling pin

Directions:

1. Spray the inside of 2 ramekins with cooking spray.
2. Place 2 flat pieces of bread into each ramekin. Add the ham slice pieces into each ramekin.
3. Crack an egg in each ramekin, then sprinkle with cheese. Season with salt and pepper.
4. Place the ramekins into the air fryer at 300°F for 15 minutes.
5. Serve warm.

Nutrition:

- Calories: 162
- Total Fat: 8 g
- Carbs: 10 g

- Protein: 11 g

23.   Breakfast Cod Nuggets

Preparation Time: 10 minutes
Cooking Time: 10 minutes
Servings: 4
Ingredients:

- 1 lb. cod

For breading:

- 2 eggs, beaten
- 2 Tbsp olive oil
- 1 cup almond flour
- ¾ cup breadcrumbs
- 1 tsp dried parsley
- Pinch sea salt
- ½ tsp black pepper

Directions:

1. Preheat the air fryer to 390°F.
2. Cut the cod into strips about 1-inch by 2-inches. Blend breadcrumbs, olive oil, salt, parsley, and pepper in a food processor.
3. In 3 separate bowls, add breadcrumbs, eggs, and flour.
4. Place each piece of fish into flour, then the eggs, and the breadcrumbs.
5. Add pieces of cod to the air fryer basket and cook for 10 minutes.
6. Serve warm.

Nutrition:

- Calories: 213
- Total Fat: 12.6 g
- Carbs: 9.2 g
- Protein: 13.4 g

24.   Vegetable Egg Pancake

Preparation Time: 10 minutes
Cooking Time: 15 minutes
Servings: 2
Ingredients:

- 1 cup almond flour
- ½ cup milk
- 1 Tbsp parmesan cheese, grated
- 3 eggs
- 1 potato, grated
- 1 beet, peeled and grated
- 1 carrot, grated
- 1 zucchini, grated
- 1 Tbsp olive oil
- ¼ tsp nutmeg
- 1 tsp onion powder

- 1 tsp garlic powder
- ½ tsp black pepper

Directions:
1. Preheat your air fryer to 390°F.
2. Mix the zucchini, potato, beet, carrot, eggs, milk, almond flour, and parmesan in a bowl.
3. Place olive oil into an oven-safe dish.
4. Form patties with the vegetable mix and flatten them to form patties.
5. Place patties into an oven-safe dish and cook in the air fryer for 15 minutes.
6. Serve with sliced tomatoes, sour cream, and toast.

Nutrition:
- Calories: 223
- Total Fat: 11.2 g
- Carbs: 10.3 g
- Proteins: 13.4 g

25.   Oriental Omelet

Preparation Time: 10 minutes
Cooking Time: 12 minutes
Servings: 1

Ingredients:
- ½ cup fresh Shimeji mushrooms, sliced
- 2 eggs, whisked
- Salt and pepper, to taste
- 1 clove garlic, minced
- A handful of sliced tofu
- 2 Tbsp onion, finely chopped
- Cooking spray

Directions:
1. Spray the baking dish with cooking spray.
2. Add onions and garlic. Air fry in the preheated air fryer at 355°F for 4 minutes.
3. Place the tofu and mushrooms over the onions and add salt and pepper to taste.
4. Whisk the eggs and pour them over tofu and mushrooms.
5. Air fry again for 20 minutes.
6. Serve warm.

Nutrition:
- Calories: 210
- Total Fat: 11.2 g
- Carbs: 8.6 g
- Protein: 12.2 g

26.   Crispy Breakfast Avocado Fries

Preparation Time: 10 minutes
Cooking Time: 8 minutes
Servings: 2

Ingredients:
- 2 eggs, beaten
- 2 large avocados, peeled, pitted, cut into 8 slices each
- ¼ tsp pepper
- ½ tsp cayenne pepper
- Salt, to taste
- ½ a lemon, Juice
- ½ cup whole-wheat flour
- 1 cup whole-wheat breadcrumbs
- Greek yogurt to serve

Directions:
1. Add flour, salt, pepper, and cayenne pepper to bowl and mix. Add bread crumbs into another bowl. Beat eggs in a third bowl.
2. First, dredge the avocado slices in the flour mixture.
3. Next, dip them into the egg mixture, and finally dredge them in the breadcrumbs.
4. Place avocado fries into the air fryer basket.
5. Preheat the air fryer to 390°F.
6. Place the air fryer basket into the air fryer and cook for 6 minutes.
7. When cook time is completed, transfer the avocado fries onto a serving platter.
8. Sprinkle with lemon juice and serve with Greek yogurt.

Nutrition:
- Calories: 272
- Total Fat: 13.4 g
- Carbs: 11.2 g
- Protein: 15.4 g

27.   Cheese and Egg Breakfast Sandwich

Preparation Time: 10 minutes
Cooking Time: 6 minutes
Servings: 1

Ingredients:
- 1–2 eggs
- 1–2 slices cheddar or Swiss cheese
- A bit butter
- 1 roll sliced in half (your choice, Kaiser Bun, English muffin, etc.)

Directions:
1. Butter your sliced roll on both sides.
2. Place the eggs in an oven-safe dish and whisk. Add seasoning if you wish, such as dill, chives, oregano, and salt.
3. Place the egg dish, roll, and cheese into the air fryer.

4. Make assured the buttered sides of the roll are in front of upwards. Set the air fryer to 390°F with a cook time of 6 minutes.
5. Remove the ingredients when cook time is completed by the air fryer.
6. Place the egg and cheese between the pieces of roll and serve warm.
7. You might like to try adding slices of avocado and tomatoes to this breakfast sandwich!

Nutrition:
- Calories: 212
- Total Fat: 11.2 g
- Carbs: 9.3 g
- Protein: 12.4 g

28.   Baked Mini Quiche

Preparation Time: 10 minutes
Cooking Time: 15 minutes
Servings: 2
Ingredients:
- 2 eggs
- 1 large yellow onion, diced
- 1 ¾ cups whole-wheat flour
- 1 ½ cups spinach, chopped
- ¾ cup cottage cheese
- Salt and black pepper, to taste
- 2 Tbsp olive oil
- ¾ cup butter
- ¼ cup milk

Directions:
1. Preheat the air fryer to 355°F. Add the flour, butter, salt, and milk to the bowl and knead the dough until smooth and refrigerate for 15 minutes.
2. Abode a frying pan over medium heat and add the oil to it.
3. When the oil is heated, add the onions into the pan and sauté them. Introduce spinach to the pan and cook until it wilts.
4. Drain the excess moisture from spinach. Whisk the eggs together and add cheese to the bowl, and mix.
5. Take the dough out of the fridge and divide it into eight equal parts. Roll the dough into a ball that will fit into the bottom of the quiche mound. Place the rolled dough into molds. Place the spinach filling over the dough.
6. Place molds into air fryer basket and place basket inside of air fryer and cook for 15 minutes. Remove quiche from molds and serve warm or cold.

Nutrition:
- Calories: 262
- Total Fat: 8.2 g
- Carbs: 7.3 g
- Protein: 9.5 g

29.   Peanut Butter and Banana Breakfast Sandwich

Preparation Time: 10 minutes
Cooking Time: 6 minutes
Servings: 1
Ingredients:
- 2 slices whole-wheat bread
- 1 tsp sugar-free maple syrup
- 1 sliced banana
- 2 Tbsp peanut butter

Directions:
1. Evenly coat both sides of the slices of bread with peanut butter.
2. Add the sliced banana and drizzle with some sugar-free maple syrup.
3. Heat in the air fryer to 330°F for 6 minutes.
4. Serve warm.

Nutrition:
- Calories: 211
- Total Fat: 8.2 g
- Carbs: 6.3 g
- Protein: 11.2 g

30.   Eggs and Cocotte on Toast

Preparation Time: 10 minutes
Cooking Time: 15 minutes
Servings: 2
Ingredients:
- 1/8 tsp black pepper
- ¼ tsp salt
- ½ tsp Italian seasoning
- ¼ tsp balsamic vinegar
- ¼ tsp sugar-free maple syrup
- 1 cup sausages, chopped into small pieces
- 2 eggs
- 2 slices whole-wheat toast
- 3 Tbsp cheddar cheese, shredded
- 6 slices tomatoes
- Cooking spray
- A little mayonnaise to serve

Directions:
1. Spray a baking dish with cooking spray. Place the bread slices at the bottom of the dish.

2. Sprinkle the sausages over the bread. Lay the tomatoes over it. Sprinkle the top with cheese.
3. Beat the eggs, and then pour over the top of bread slices. Drizzle vinegar and maple syrup over eggs.
4. Flavor with Italian seasoning, salt, and pepper, then sprinkle some more cheese on top.
5. Place the baking dish in the air fryer basket that should be preheated at 320°F and cooked for 10 minutes.
6. Remove from the air fryer and add a touch of mayonnaise and serve.

Nutrition:
- Calories: 232
- Total Fat: 7.4 g
- Carbs: 6.3 g
- Protein: 14.2 g

31. Breakfast Frittata

Preparation Time: 10 minutes
Cooking Time: 15 minutes
Servings: 3

Ingredients:
- 6 eggs
- 8 cherry tomatoes, halved
- 2 Tbsp parmesan cheese, shredded
- 1 Italian sausage, diced
- Salt and pepper, to taste

Directions:
1. Preheat your air fryer to 355°F. Add the tomatoes and sausage to the baking dish.
2. Place the baking dish into the air fryer and cook for 5 minutes.
3. Meanwhile, add eggs, salt, pepper, cheese, and oil into a mixing bowl, and whisk well.
4. Remove the baking dish from the air fryer and pour the egg mixture on top, spreading evenly.
5. Place the dish back into the air fryer and bake for additional 5 minutes.
6. Remove from the air fryer and slice into wedges and serve.

Nutrition:
- Calories: 273
- Total Fat: 8.2 g
- Carbs: 7 g
- Protein: 14.2 g

32. Morning Mini Cheeseburger Sliders

Preparation Time: 10 minutes
Cooking Time: 10 minutes
Servings: 6

Ingredients:
- 1 lb. ground beef
- 6 slices cheddar cheese
- 6 dinner rolls
- Salt and black pepper, to taste

Directions:
1. Preheat your air fryer to 390°F.
2. Form 6 beef patties, each about 2.5 oz., and season with salt and black pepper.
3. Add the burger patties to the cooking basket and cook them for 10minutes.
4. Remove the burger patties from the air fryer, place the cheese on top of burgers, and return to the air fryer and cook for another minute.
5. Remove and put burgers on dinner rolls and serve warm.

Nutrition:
- Calories: 262
- Total Fat: 9.4 g
- Carbs: 8.2 g
- Protein: 16.2 g

33. Avocado and Blueberry Muffins

Preparation Time: 10 minutes
Cooking Time: 15 minutes
Servings: 12

Ingredients:
- 2 eggs
- 1 cup blueberries
- 2 cups almond flour
- 1 tsp baking soda
- 1/8 tsp salt
- 2 ripe avocados, peeled, pitted, mashed
- 2 Tbsp liquid Stevia
- 1 cup plain Greek yogurt
- 1 tsp vanilla extract

For the streusel topping:
- 2 Tbsp Truvia sweetener
- 4 Tbsp butter, softened
- 4 Tbsp almond flour

Directions:
1. Make the streusel topping by mixing Truvia, flour, and butter until you form a crumbly mixture. Place this mixture in the freezer for a while.
2. Meanwhile, make the muffins by sifting together flour, baking powder, baking soda, and salt, and set aside. Add avocados and liquid Stevia to a bowl and mix well. Adding in one egg at a time, continue to beat. Add the vanilla extract and yogurt and beat again.

3. Add in flour mixture a bit at a time and mix well. Add the blueberries into the mixture and gently fold them in. Pour the batter into greased muffin cups, then add the mixture until they are half-full.
4. Sprinkle the streusel topping mixture on top of the muffin mixture and place muffin cups in the air fryer basket.
5. Bake in the preheated air fryer at 355°F for 10 minutes. Remove the muffin cups from the air fryer and allow them to cool. Cool completely, then serve.

Nutrition:
- Calories: 202
- Total Fat: 9.2 g
- Carbs: 7.2 g
- Protein: 6.3 g

34.   Cheese Omelette

Preparation Time: 10 minutes
Cooking Time: 15 minutes
Servings: 2

Ingredients:
- 3 eggs
- 1 large yellow onion, diced
- 2 Tbsp cheddar cheese, shredded
- ½ tsp soy sauce
- Salt and pepper, to taste
- Olive oil cooking spray

Directions:
1. In a container, whisk together eggs, soy sauce, pepper, and salt. Spray with olive oil cooking spray a small pan that will fit inside of your air fryer.
2. Transfer onions to the pan and spread them around. Air fry onions for 7 minutes.
3. Pour the beaten egg mixture over the cooked onions and sprinkle the top with shredded cheese.
4. Take back into the air fryer and cook for 6 minutes more.
5. Remove from the air fryer and serve Omelette with toasted multi-grain bread.

Nutrition:
- Calories: 232
- Total Fat: 8.2 g
- Carbs: 6.2 g
- Protein: 12.3 g

35.   Cheese and Mushroom Frittata

Preparation Time: 8–10 minutes
Cooking Time: 15 minutes
Servings: 4

Ingredients:
- 4 cups Button Mushrooms, cut into ¼-inch slices
- 1 Large Red Onion, cut into ¼-inch slices
- 2 Tbsp Olive Oil
- 1 tsp Garlic, minced
- 6 Eggs
- Salt, to taste
- Ground Black Pepper, to taste
- 6 Tbsp Feta Cheese

Directions:
1. Put the button mushrooms, onions, and garlic in a pan with a Tbsp of olive oil, and sauté over medium heat for 5 minutes.
2. Transfer to a kitchen towel to dry and cool.
3. Warm up the Air Fryer to 330°F.
4. Place eggs in a bowl and whisk lightly. Flavor with salt and pepper, and then whisk well.
5. Brush the baking accessory with olive oil
6. Place sautéed onions and mushrooms in the baking accessory, crumble the feta cheese over it, and then pour the eggs on top.
7. Cook for 20 minutes or until a skewer stuck in the middle of the frittata comes out clean.
8. Serve warm.
9. Enjoy!

Nutrition:
- Calories: 232
- Total Fat: 8.2 g
- Carbs: 6.2 g
- Protein: 12.3 g

36.   Bagels

Preparation Time: 20 minutes
Cooking Time: 15 minutes
Servings: 12

Ingredients:
- ½ lb. flour
- 1 tsp Active dry yeast
- 1 tsp Brown sugar
- ½ cup lukewarm water
- 2 Tbsp butter softened
- 1 tsp salt
- 1 large egg

Directions:
1. Liquefy the yeast and sugar in the warm water. Let rest for 5 minutes.
2. Add the remaining ingredients and mix until sticky dough forms. Cover and let rest for 40 minutes.
3. Massage the dough on a lightly floured surface and divide it into 5 large balls. Let rest for 4 minutes.
4. Preheat air fryer to 360°F.

5. Flatted the dough balls and make a hole in the center of each. Arrange the bagels on a baking sheet lined with parchment paper — Bake for 20 minutes.
6. Enjoy!

Nutrition:
- Calories: 232
- Total Fat: 8.2 g
- Carbs: 6.2 g
- Protein: 12.3 g

37.   Vegetarian Omelet

Preparation Time: 16 minutes
Cooking Time: 15 minutes
Servings: 2

Ingredients:
- 8 oz. spinach leaves
- 3 Spring Onions, cut into 1-inch slices
- ½ Red Bull Pepper, cut into 1-inch cubes
- 1 cup Button Mushrooms, cut into ¼-inch slices
- ½ tsp. Ground Turmeric
- 1 tsp. thyme
- 1 tsp. Kala Namak Salt
- ½ tsp. Ground Black Pepper
- 1 tsp. Minced Garlic
- 3 Tbsp. Olive Oil (extra virgin)
- 2 Tbsp. Butter
- 1 cup Chickpea Flour
- 1 cup Water

Directions:
1. In a bowl, place spring onions, bell peppers, mushrooms, turmeric, thyme, Kala Namak salt, ground black pepper, minced garlic, and 2 Tbsp. of olive oil. Toss well to combine.
2. Heat a sauté pan over medium-high heat and tip in the vegetable mixture.
3. Sauté for 3 minutes, frequently tossing.
4. Add spinach and butter to the pan, and sauté for another 3 minutes, frequently tossing.
5. Remove from the heat and set aside until needed.
6. Place the chickpea flour and water in a bowl, and whisk to smooth batter.
7. Grease the Air Fryer accessory with olive oil and pour in the batter.
8. Cook for 3 minutes at 390°F. Flip and cook for another 3 minutes.
9. Transfer fried Omelette on a serving plate and top with sautéed vegetables.
10. Serve with salsa on the side.
11. Enjoy!

Nutrition:
- Calories: 232

- Total Fat: 8.2 g
- Carbs: 6.2 g
- Protein: 12.3 g

38.   Bacon and Cheese Rolls

Preparation Time: 8–10 minutes
Cooking Time: 15 minutes
Servings: 4

Ingredients:
- 1 lb. Cheddar Cheese, grated
- 1 lb. Bacon Rashers
- 1 8 oz. can Pillsbury Crescent Dough

Directions:
1. Warm up the Air Fryer to 330°F.
2. Cut the bacon rashers across into ¼ inch strips and mix with the cheddar cheese. Set aside.
3. Cut the dough sheet to 1 by 1.5 inches pieces.
4. Place an equal amount of bacon and cheese mixture on the center of the dough pieces and pinch corners together to enclose stuffing.
5. Transfer the parcels in the Air Fry basket and bake for 7 minutes at 330°F.
6. Increase the temperature to 390°F and bake for another 3 minutes.
7. Serve warm.
8. Enjoy!

Nutrition:
- Calories: 232
- Total Fat: 8.2 g
- Carbs: 6.2 g
- Protein: 12.3 g

39.   Meatballs and Creamy Potatoes

Preparation Time: 45–50 minutes
Cooking Time: 15 minutes
Servings: 4–6

Ingredients:
- 12 oz. Lean Ground Beef
- 1 medium Onion, finely chopped
- 1 Tbsp Parsley Leaves, finely chopped
- ½ Tbsp Fresh Thyme Leaves
- ½ tsp Minced Garlic
- 2 Tbsp Olive Oil
- 1 tsp Salt
- 1 tsp Ground Black Pepper
- 1 Enormous Egg
- 3 Tbsp Bread Crumbs
- 1 cup Half & Half, or ½ cup Whole Milk and ½ cup Cream mixed
- 7 Medium Russet Potatoes

- ½ tsp Ground Nutmeg
- ½ cup Grated Gruyere Cheese

Directions:

1. Place the ground beef, onions, parsley, thyme, garlic, olive oil, salt and pepper, egg, and breadcrumbs in a bowl, and mix well. Place in refrigerator until needed.
2. In another bowl, place half & half and nutmeg, and whisk to combine.
3. Peel and wash potatoes, and then slice them thinly, 1/8 to 1/5 of an inch, if needed, to use a mandolin.
4. Warm up the Air Fryer to 390°F.
5. Place potato slices in a bowl with half & half and toss to coat well.
6. Layer the potato slices in an Air Fryer baking accessory and pour over the leftover half & half.
7. Bake for 25 minutes at 390°F.
8. Meanwhile, take the meat mixture out of the fridge and shape it into inch and half balls.
9. When potatoes are cooked, place meatballs on top of them in one layer and cover with the grated Gruyere.
10. Cook for another 10 minutes.
11. Enjoy!

Nutrition:

- Calories: 232
- Total Fat: 8.2 g
- Carbs: 6.2 g
- Protein: 12.3 g

40.   Sweet Potato Fritters

Preparation Time: 6–7 minutes
Cooking Time: 15 minutes
Servings: 4

Ingredients:

- 1 can Sweet Potato Puree, 15 oz.
- ½ tsp Minced Garlic
- ½ cup Frozen Spinach, thawed, finely chopped, and drained well
- 1 Large Leek, minced
- 1 serving Flax Egg
- ¼ cup Almond Flour
- ¼ tsp Sweet Paprika Flakes
- 1 tsp Kosher Salt
- ½ tsp Ground White Pepper

Directions:

1. Heat the Air Fryer to 330°F.
2. Place all ingredients in a bowl and mix all well.
3. Divide into 16 balls and flatten each to only an-inch-thick patty.
4. Place patties in the Air Fryer basket and cook for two minutes at 330°F.
5. Flip and cook for 2 more minutes.
6. If needed, cook in batches.
7. Enjoy!

Nutrition:

- Calories: 232
- Total Fat: 8.2 g
- Carbs: 6.2 g
- Protein: 12.3 g

Chapter 4.   Appetizer and Sides Recipes

41.   Garlic Kale Chips

Preparation Time: 6–7 minutes
Cooking Time: 10 minutes
Servings: 2
Ingredients:

- 1 Tbsp yeast flakes
- Sea salt, to taste
- 1 tsp vegan seasoning
- 4 cups packed kale
- 2 Tbsp olive oil
- 1 tsp garlic, minced

Directions:

1. In a bowl, place the oil, kale, garlic, and ranch seasoning pieces. Add the yeast and mix well.
2. Dump the coated kale into the air fryer basket and cook at 375°F for 5 minutes.
3. Shake after 3 minutes and serve.

Nutrition:

- Calories: 50
- Total Fat: 1.9 g
- Carbs: 10 g
- Protein: 46 g

42.   Garlic Salmon Balls

Preparation Time: 6–7 minutes
Cooking Time: 15 minutes
Servings: 2
Ingredients:

- 6 oz. tinned salmon
- 1 large egg
- 3 Tbsp olive oil
- 5 Tbsp wheat germ
- ½ tsp garlic powder
- 1 Tbsp dill, fresh, chopped
- 4 Tbsp spring onion, diced
- 4 Tbsp celery, diced

Directions:

1. Preheat your air fryer to 370°F.
2. In a large bowl, mix the salmon, egg, celery, onion, dill, and garlic.
3. Shape the mixture into golf ball size balls and roll them in the wheat germ.
4. In a small pan, warm olive oil over medium-low heat.
5. Add the salmon balls and slowly flatten them.

6. Transfer them to your air fryer and cook for 10 minutes.

Nutrition:

- Calories: 219
- Total Fat: 7.7 g
- Carbs: 14.8 g
- Protein: 23.1 g

43.   Onion Rings

Preparation Time: 7 minutes
Cooking Time: 10 minutes
Servings: 3
Ingredients:

- 1 onion, cut into slices, then separate into rings
- 1 ½ cups almond flour
- ¾ cup pork rinds
- 1 cup milk
- 1 egg
- 1 Tbsp baking powder
- ½ tsp salt

Directions:

1. Preheat your air fryer for 10 minutes.
2. Cut onion into slices, then separate into rings. In a container, introduce the flour, baking powder, and salt.
3. Whisk the eggs and the milk, then combines with flour.
4. Gently dip the floured onion rings into the batter to coat them.
5. Spread the pork rinds on a plate and dredge the rings in the crumbs.
6. Place the onion rings in your air fryer and cook for 10 minutes at 360°F.

Nutrition:

- Calories: 304
- Total Fat: 18 g
- Carbs: 31 g
- Protein: 38 g

44.   Crispy Eggplant Fries

Preparation Time: 7 minutes
Cooking Time: 12 minutes
Servings: 3
Ingredients:

- 2 eggplants
- ¼ cup olive oil

- ¼ cup almond flour
- ½ cup water

Directions:
1. Preheat your air fryer to 390°F.
2. Cut the eggplants into half-inch slices. In a mixing bowl, mix the flour, olive oil, water, and eggplants. Slowly coat the eggplants.
3. Add eggplants to the air fryer and cook for 12 minutes.
4. Serve with yogurt or tomato sauce.

Nutrition:
- Calories: 103
- Total Fat: 7.3 g
- Carbs: 12.3 g
- Protein: 1.9 g

45.   Charred Bell Peppers

Preparation Time: 7 minutes
Cooking Time: 4 minutes
Servings: 3

Ingredients:
- 20 bell peppers, sliced and seeded
- 1 tsp olive oil
- 1 pinch sea salt
- 1 lemon

Directions:
1. Preheat your air fryer to 390°F. Sprinkle the peppers with oil and salt.
2. Cook the peppers in the air fryer for 4 minutes.
3. Place peppers in a large bowl and squeeze lemon juice over the top.
4. Season with salt and pepper.

Nutrition:
- Calories: 30
- Total Fat: 0.25 g
- Carbs: 6.91 g
- Protein: 1.28 g

46.   Garlic Tomatoes

Preparation Time: 7 minutes
Cooking Time: 15 minutes
Servings: 4

Ingredients:
- 3 Tbsp vinegar
- ½ tsp thyme, dried
- 4 tomatoes
- 1 Tbsp olive oil
- Salt and black pepper, to taste
- 1 clove garlic, minced

Directions:
1. Preheat your air fryer to 390°F. Cut the tomatoes into halves and remove the seeds.
2. Place them in a big bowl and toss them with oil, salt, pepper, garlic, and thyme.
3. Place them into the air fryer and cook for 15 minutes.
4. Drizzle with vinegar and serve.

Nutrition:
- Calories: 28.9
- Total Fat: 2.4 g
- Carbs: 2.0 g
- Protein: 0.4 g

47.   Mushroom Stew

Preparation Time: 7 minutes
Cooking Time: 1 hour and 22 minutes
Servings: 6

Ingredients:
- 1 lb. chicken, cubed, boneless, skinless
- 2 Tbsp canola oil
- 1 lb. Fresh mushrooms, sliced
- 1 Tbsp thyme, dried
- ¾ cup water
- 2 Tbsp tomato paste
- 3 large tomatoes, chopped
- 4 cloves garlic, minced
- 1 cup green peppers, sliced
- 3 cups zucchini, diced
- 1 large onion, diced
- 1 Tbsp basil
- 1 Tbsp marjoram
- 1 Tbsp oregano

Directions:
1. Cut the chicken into cubes. Position them in the air fryer basket and pour olive oil over them.
2. Add mushrooms, zucchini, onion, and green pepper. Mix and add in garlic, cook for 2 minutes, then add in tomato paste, water, and seasonings.
3. Lock the air fryer and cook the stew for 50 minutes.
4. Set the heat to 340°F and cook for an additional 20 minutes.
5. Remove from air fryer and transfer into a large pan.
6. Add in a bit of water and simmer for 10 minutes.

Nutrition:
- Calories: 53
- Total Fat: 3.3 g
- Carbs: 4.9 g
- Protein: 2.3 g

48.   Cheese and Onion Nuggets

Preparation Time: 7 minutes
Cooking Time: 12 minutes
Servings: 4
Ingredients:

- 7 oz. Edam cheese, grated
- 2 spring onions, diced
- 1 egg, beaten
- 1 Tbsp coconut oil
- 1 Tbsp thyme, dried
- Salt and pepper, to taste

Directions:

1. Mix the onion, cheese, coconut oil, salt, pepper, and thyme in a bowl.
2. Make 8 small balls and place the cheese in the center.
3. Put them in the fridge for about an hour.
4. With a pastry brush, carefully brush beaten egg over the nuggets.
5. Cook for 12 minutes in the air fryer at 350 Fahrenheit.

Nutrition:

- Calories: 227
- Total Fat: 17.3 g
- Carbs: 4.5 g
- Protein: 14.2 g

49.   Spiced Nuts

Preparation Time: 7 minutes
Cooking Time: 10 minutes
Servings: 3 cups
Ingredients:

- 1 cup almonds
- 1 cup pecan halves
- 1 cup cashews
- 1 egg white, beaten
- ½ tsp cinnamon, ground
- Pinch cayenne pepper
- ¼ tsp cloves, ground
- Dash salt

Directions:

1. Combine the egg white with spices.
2. Preheat your air fryer to 300°F. Toss the nuts in the spiced mixture.
3. Cook for 25 minutes, stirring several times throughout cooking time.

Nutrition:

- Calories: 88.4
- Total Fat: 7.6 g
- Carbs: 3.9 g

- Protein: 2.5 g

50.   Keto French fries

Preparation Time: 7 minutes
Cooking Time: 20 minutes
Servings: 4
Ingredients:

- 1 large rutabaga, peeled, cut into spears about ¼ inch wide
- Salt and pepper, to taste
- ½ tsp paprika
- 2 Tbsp coconut oil

Directions:

1. Preheat your air fryer to 450°F.
2. Mix the oil, paprika, salt, and pepper.
3. Pour the oil mixture over the fries, making sure all pieces are well coated.
4. Cook in the air fryer for 20 minutes or until crispy.

Nutrition:

- Calories: 113
- Total Fat: 7.2 g
- Carbs: 12.5 g
- Protein: 1.9 g

51.   Fried Garlic Green Tomatoes

Preparation Time: 7 minutes
Cooking Time: 12 minutes
Servings: 2
Ingredients:

- 3 green tomatoes, sliced
- ½ cup almond flour
- 2 eggs, beaten
- Salt and pepper, to taste
- 1 tsp garlic, minced

Directions:

1. Season the tomatoes with salt, garlic, and pepper.
2. Preheat your air fryer to 400°F.
3. Dip the tomatoes first in flour, then in the egg mixture. Spray the tomato rounds with olive oil and place them in the air fryer basket.
4. Cook for 8 minutes, then flip over and cook for additional 4 minutes.
5. Serve with zero-carb mayonnaise.

Nutrition:

- Calories: 123
- Total Fat: 3.9 g
- Carbs: 16 g
- Protein: 8.4 g

52. Garlic Cauliflower Tots

Preparation Time: 7 minutes
Cooking Time: 20 minutes
Servings: 6

Ingredients:

- 1 crown cauliflower, chopped in a food processor
- ½ cup parmesan cheese, grated
- Salt and pepper, to taste
- ¼ cup almond flour
- 2 eggs
- 1 tsp garlic, minced

Directions:

1. Mix all the ingredients. Shape into tots and spray with olive oil.
2. Preheat your air fryer to 400°F.
3. Cook for 10 minutes on each side.

Nutrition:

- Calories: 18
- Total Fat: 0.6 g
- Carbs: 1.3 g
- Protein: 1.8 g

53. Green Onions and Parmesan Tomatoes

Preparation Time: 7 minutes
Cooking Time: 15 minutes
Servings: 4

Ingredients:

- 4 large tomatoes, cut into slices
- 1 Tbsp olive oil
- Salt and pepper, to taste
- ½ tsp thyme, dried
- 2 garlic cloves, minced
- 2 green onions, finely chopped
- ½ cup parmesan, freshly grated

Directions:

1. Preheat your air fryer to 390°F.
2. Coat the tomato slices with olive oil, season with garlic, thyme, salt, and pepper.
3. Top with parmesan and chopped green onions.
4. Place tomatoes in the air fryer and cook for 15 minutes.
5. Serve on top of crostini or any meat, poultry, or fish.

Nutrition:

- Calories: 69
- Total Fat: 3.9 g
- Carbs: 69 g
- Protein: 1.6 g

54. Green Bell Peppers with Cauliflower Stuffing

Preparation Time: 7 minutes
Cooking Time: 20 minutes
Servings: 4

Ingredients:

- 4 green bell peppers, top cut, deseeded
- 1 tsp lemon juice
- 2 Tbsp coriander leaves, finely chopped
- 2 green chilies, finely chopped
- 2 cups cauliflower, cooked and mashed
- 2 onions, finely chopped
- 1 tsp cumin seeds
- ¼ tsp turmeric powder
- ¼ tsp chili powder
- ¼ tsp garam masala
- Salt, to taste
- Olive oil as needed

Directions:

1. In a saucepan, heat the oil and sauté the chilies, onion, and cumin seeds.
2. Add the rest of the ingredients except the bell peppers and mix well.
3. Preheat your air fryer to 390°F for 10 minutes.
4. Brush the green bell peppers with olive oil, inside and out, and stuff each pepper with cauliflower mixture.
5. Place them into the air fryer and grill for 10 minutes.

Nutrition:

- Calories: 257
- Total Fat: 4.0 g
- Carbs: 44.8 g
- Protein: 12.3 g

55. Cheesy Chickpea and Courgette Burgers

Preparation Time: 7 minutes
Cooking Time: 10 minutes
Servings: 4

Ingredients:

- 1 can chickpeas (drained
- 3 Tbsp coriander
- 1 oz. cheddar cheese, shredded
- 2 eggs, beaten
- 1 tsp garlic puree
- 1 zucchini (spiralizer
- 1 red onion, diced
- 1 tsp chili powder
- 1 tsp mixed spice
- Salt and pepper, to taste

- 1 tsp cumin

Directions:
1. Mix your ingredients in a mixing bowl.
2. Shape portions of the mixture into burgers.
3. Place in the air fryer at 300°F for 15 minutes.

Nutrition:
- Calories: 184.8
- Total Fat: 10.1 g,
- Carbs: 18.4 g
- Protein: 13.2 g

56. Spicy Sweet Potatoes

Preparation Time: 7 minutes
Cooking Time: 23 minutes
Servings: 4

Ingredients:
- 3 sweet potatoes, peeled and chopped into chips
- 1 tsp chili powder
- 1 tsp paprika
- 2 Tbsp olive oil
- 1 Tbsp red wine vinegar
- 1 tomato, thinly sliced
- ½ cup tomato sauce
- 1 onion, peeled and diced
- Salt and pepper, to taste
- 1 tsp rosemary
- 1 tsp oregano
- 1 tsp mixed spice
- 2 tsp thyme
- 2 tsp coriander

Directions:
1. Toss the chips in a bowl with olive oil.
2. Add to the air fryer and cook for 15 minutes at 360°F.
3. Mix the remaining ingredients in a baking dish.
4. Place the sauce in the air fryer for 8 minutes.
5. Toss the potatoes in the sauce and serve warm.

Nutrition:
- Calories: 303
- Total Fat: 5 g
- Carbs: 57 g
- Protein: 8 g

57. Olive, Cheese, and Broccoli

Preparation Time: 7 minutes
Cooking Time: 15 minutes
Servings: 4

Ingredients:
- 2 lbs. broccoli florets

- 2 Tbsp olive oil
- ¼ cup parmesan cheese shaved
- 2 tsp lemon zest, grated
- 1/3 cup Kalamata olives (halved, pitted
- ½ tsp ground black pepper
- 1 tsp sea salt

Directions:
1. Boil the water in a pan over medium heat and cook the broccoli for about 4 minutes. Drain.
2. Fling the broccoli with salt, pepper, and olive oil in a bowl.
3. Place in the air fryer and cook at 400°F for 15 minutes. Toss twice during cook time.
4. Move to a dish and toss with lemon zest, cheese, and olives.

Nutrition:
- Calories: 214
- Total Fat: 13.45 g
- Carbs: 13.22 g
- Protein: 12.56 g

58. Veggie Mix

Preparation Time: 7 minutes
Cooking Time: 35 minutes
Servings: 4

Ingredients:
- ½ lb. carrots, peeled, cubed
- 6 tsp olive oil
- ½ tsp tarragon leaves
- ½ tsp white pepper
- Salt, to taste
- 1 lb. Yellow squash, chopped into wedges
- 1 lb. Zucchini, chopped into wedges

Directions:
1. Toss the carrots with 2 tsp of olive oil in your air fryer basket. Cook at 400°F for 5 minutes.
2. Toss in the squash and zucchini along with the rest of the oil, salt, and pepper into the air fryer.
3. Cook for additional 30 minutes, tossing twice during cook time.
4. Toss with tarragon and serve.

Nutrition:
- Calories: 162
- Total Fat: 1.2 g
- Carbs: 30.3 g
- Protein: 7.5 g

59.	Garlic and Cheese Potatoes

Preparation Time: 7 minutes
Cooking Time: 40 minutes
Servings: 4

Ingredients:

- 4 Idaho baking potatoes, halved
- 1 Tbsp garlic powder
- Salt, to taste
- ½ cup cheddar cheese, shredded
- 1 tsp parsley

Directions:

1. Toss all your ingredients in a bowl except cheese.
2. Place potatoes in a baking dish and sprinkle cheese over top of them.
3. Cook for 40 minutes at 390°F.

Nutrition:

- Calories: 498
- Total Fat: 19.09 g
- Carbs: 67.27 g
- Protein: 16.5 g

60.	Garlic Baby Potatoes

Preparation Time: 7 minutes
Cooking Time: 10 minutes
Servings: 2

Ingredients:

- 8 oz. boiled baby potatoes
- ½ tsp sesame seeds
- Red chili powder, to taste
- Salt and pepper, to taste
- ½ tsp garlic paste
- ¼ tsp coriander seeds, dry roasted
- ¼ tsp cumin seeds, dry roasted
- ½ cup fresh cream

Directions:

1. Grind the coriander and cumin seeds to form a powder. Toss all the ingredients in a baking dish except the cream.
2. Preheat your air fryer for 5 minutes at 360°F. Cook potatoes for 5 minutes.
3. Mix in cream and air fry for an additional 5 minutes.
4. Garnish with sesame seeds.

Nutrition:

- Calories: 498
- Total Fat: 19.09 g
- Carbs: 67.27 g
- Protein: 16.5 g

Chapter 5.   Meat Recipes

61.   Beef Korma Curry

Preparation Time: 10 minutes
Cooking Time: 17–20 minutes
Servings: 4
Ingredients:

- 1 lb. (454 g) sirloin steak, sliced
- ½ cup yogurt
- 1 Tbsp curry powder
- 1 Tbsp olive oil
- 1 onion, chopped
- 2 cloves garlic, minced
- 1 tomato, diced
- ½ cup frozen baby peas, thawed

Directions:

1. In a medium bowl, combine the steak, yogurt, and curry powder. Stir and set aside.
2. In a metal bowl, combine the olive oil, onion, and garlic. Bake at 350°F (177°C) for 3 to 4 minutes or until crisp and tender.
3. Add the steak along with the yogurt and the diced tomato. Bake for 12 to 13 minutes or until the steak is almost tender.
4. Stir in the peas and bake for 2 to 3 minutes or until hot.

Nutrition:

- Calories: 299
- Fat: 11 g
- Protein: 38 g
- Carbs: 9 g
- Fiber: 2 g
- Sugar: 3 g
- Sodium: 100 mg

62.   Chicken Fried Steak

Preparation Time: 15 minutes
Cooking Time: 12–16 minutes
Servings: 4
Ingredients:

- 4 (6 oz./170 g) beef cube steaks
- ½ cup buttermilk
- 1 cup flour
- 2 tsp paprika
- 1 tsp garlic salt
- 1 egg
- 1 cup soft bread crumbs
- 2 Tbsp olive oil

Directions:

1. Place the cube steaks on a plate or cutting board and gently lb. until they are slightly thinner. Set aside.
2. In a shallow bowl, combine the buttermilk, flour, paprika, garlic salt, and egg until combined.
3. On a plate, combine the bread crumbs and olive oil and mix well.
4. Dip the steaks into the buttermilk batter to coat and let sit on a plate for 5 minutes.
5. Dredge the steaks in the bread crumbs. Pat the crumbs onto both sides to coat the steaks thoroughly.
6. Air fry the steaks at 350°F (177°C) for 12 to 16 minutes or until the meat reaches 160°F (71°C) on a meat thermometer and the coating is brown and crisp. You can serve this with heated beef gravy.

Nutrition:

- Calories: 631
- Fat: 21 g
- Protein: 61 g
- Carbs: 46 g
- Fiber: 2 g
- Sugar: 3 g
- Sodium: 358 mg

63.   Lemon Greek Beef and Vegetables

Preparation Time: 10 minutes
Cooking Time: 9–19 minutes
Servings: 4
Ingredients:

- ½ lb. (227 g) 96% lean ground beef
- 2 medium tomatoes, chopped
- 1 onion, chopped
- 2 garlic cloves, minced
- 2 cups fresh baby spinach
- 2 Tbsp freshly squeezed lemon juice
- 1/3 cup low-sodium beef broth
- 2 Tbsp crumbled low-sodium feta cheese

Directions:

1. In a baking pan, crumble the beef. Place it in the air fryer basket. Air fry at 370°F (188°C) for 3 to 7 minutes, stirring once during cooking until browned. Drain off any fat or liquid.
2. Swell the tomatoes, onion, and garlic into the pan. Air fry for 4 to 8 minutes more, or until the onion is tender.

3. Add the spinach, lemon juice, and beef broth.
4. Air fry for 2 to 4 minutes more, or until the spinach is wilted.
5. Sprinkle with the feta cheese and serve immediately.

Nutrition:
- Calories: 98
- Fat: 1 g
- Protein: 15 g
- Carbs: 5 g
- Fiber: 1 g
- Sugar: 2 g
- Sodium: 123 mg

64. Country-Style Pork Ribs

Preparation Time: 5 minutes
Cooking Time: 20–25 minutes
Servings: 4

Ingredients:
- 12 country-style pork ribs, trimmed of excess fat
- 2 Tbsp cornstarch
- 2 Tbsp olive oil
- 1 tsp dry mustard
- ½ tsp thyme
- ½ tsp garlic powder
- 1 tsp dried marjoram
- Pinch salt
- Freshly ground black pepper, to taste

Directions:
1. Place the ribs on a clean work surface.
2. In a small bowl, combine the cornstarch, olive oil, mustard, thyme, garlic powder, marjoram, salt, and pepper, and rub into the ribs.
3. Place the ribs in the air fryer basket and roast at 400°F (204°C) for 10 minutes.
4. Carefully turn the ribs using tongs and roast for 10 to 15 minutes or until the ribs are crisp and register an internal temperature of at least 150°F (66°C).

Nutrition:
- Calories: 579
- Fat: 44 g
- Protein: 40 g
- Carbs: 4 g
- Fiber: 0 g
- Sugar: 0 g
- Sodium: 155 mg

65. Lemon and Honey Pork Tenderloin

Preparation Time: 5 minutes
Cooking Time: 10 minutes
Servings: 4

Ingredients:
- 1 (1 lb./454 g) pork tenderloin, cut into ½-inch slices
- 1 Tbsp olive oil
- 1 Tbsp freshly squeezed lemon juice
- 1 Tbsp honey
- ½ tsp grated lemon zest
- ½ tsp dried marjoram
- Pinch salt
- Freshly ground black pepper, to taste

Directions:
1. Put the pork tenderloin slices in a medium bowl.
2. In a minor bowl, combine the olive oil, lemon juice, honey, lemon zest, marjoram, salt, and pepper. Mix.
3. Pour this marinade over the tenderloin slices and massage gently with your hand to work it into the pork.
4. Place the pork in the air fryer basket and roast at 400°F (204°C) for 10 minutes or until the pork registers at least 145°F (63°C) using a meat thermometer.

Nutrition:
- Calories: 208
- Fat: 8 g
- Protein: 30 g
- Carbs: 5 g
- Fiber: 0 g
- Sugar: 4
- Sodium: 104 mg

66. Dijon Pork Tenderloin

Preparation Time: 10 minutes
Cooking Time: 12–14 minutes
Servings: 4

Ingredients:
- 1 lb. (454 g) pork tenderloin, cut into 1-inch slices
- Pinch salt
- Freshly ground black pepper, to taste
- 2 Tbsp Dijon mustard
- 1 clove garlic, minced
- ½ tsp dried basil
- 1 cup soft bread crumbs
- 2 Tbsp olive oil

Directions:
1. Slightly lb. the pork slices until they are about ¾ inch thick. Sprinkle with salt and pepper on both sides.
2. Coat the pork with the Dijon mustard and sprinkle with the garlic and basil.

3. On a plate, combine the bread crumbs and olive oil and mix well. Coat the pork slices with the bread crumb mixture, patting, so the crumbs adhere.

4. Place the pork in the air fryer basket, leaving a little space between each piece. Air fry at 390°F (199°C) for 12 to 14 minutes or until the pork reaches at least 145°F (63°C) on a meat thermometer and the coating is crisp and brown. Serve immediately.

Nutrition:
- Calories: 336
- Fat: 13 g
- Protein: 34 g
- Carbs: 20 g
- Fiber: 2 g
- Sugar 2 g
- Sodium: 390 mg

67. Air Fryer Pork Satay

Preparation Time: 15 minutes
Cooking Time: 9–14 minutes
Servings: 4
Ingredients:
- 1 (1 lb./454 g) pork tenderloin, cut into 1½-inch cubes
- ¼ cup minced onion
- 2 garlic cloves, minced
- 1 jalapeño pepper, minced
- 2 Tbsp freshly squeezed lime juice
- 2 Tbsp coconut milk
- 2 Tbsp unsalted peanut butter
- 2 tsp curry powder

Directions:
1. In a medium bowl, mix the pork, onion, garlic, jalapeño, lime juice, coconut milk, peanut butter, and curry powder until well combined. Let position for 10 minutes at room temperature.
2. With a slotted spoon, remove the pork from the marinade. Reserve the marinade.
3. Thread the pork onto about 8 bamboo or metal skewers. Air fry at 380°F (193°C) for 9 to 14 minutes, brushing once with the reserved marinade until the pork reaches at least 145°F (63°C) on a meat thermometer. Discard any remaining marinade. Serve immediately.

Nutrition:
- Calories: 195
- Fat: 7 g
- Protein: 25 g
- Carbs: 7 g
- Fiber: 1 g

- Sugar: 3 g
- Sodium: 65 mg

68. Pork Burgers with Red Cabbage Slaw

Preparation Time: 20 minutes
Cooking Time: 7–9 minutes
Servings: 4
Ingredients:
- ½ cup Greek yogurt
- 2 Tbsp low-sodium mustard, divided
- 1 Tbsp freshly squeezed lemon juice
- ¼ cup sliced red cabbage
- ¼ cup grated carrots
- 1 lb. (454 g) lean ground pork
- ½ tsp paprika
- 1 cup mixed baby lettuce greens
- 2 small tomatoes, sliced
- 8 small low-sodium whole-wheat sandwich buns, cut in half

Directions:
1. In a small bowl, mix the yogurt, 1 Tbsp mustard, lemon juice, cabbage, and carrots; mix and refrigerate.
2. In a medium bowl, combine the pork, remaining 1 Tbsp mustard, and paprika. Form 8 small patties.
3. Lay the patties into the air fryer basket. Air fry at 400°F (204°C) for 7 to 9 minutes, or until the patties register 165°F (74°C) as tested with a meat thermometer.
4. Assemble the burgers by placing some of the lettuce greens on the bun bottom. Top with a tomato slice, the patties, and the cabbage mixture. Add the bun top and serve immediately.

Nutrition:
- Calories: 473
- Fat: 15 g
- Protein: 35 g
- Carbs: 51 g
- Fiber: 8 g
- Sugar: 8 g
- Sodium: 138 mg

69. Greek Lamb Pita Pockets

Preparation Time: 15 minutes
Cooking Time: 5–7 minutes
Servings: 4
Ingredients:
Dressing:
- 1 cup plain Greek yogurt
- 1 Tbsp lemon juice

- 1 tsp dried dill weed, crushed
- 1 tsp ground oregano
- ½ tsp salt

Meatballs:
- ½ lb. (227 g) ground lamb
- 1 Tbsp diced onion
- 1 tsp dried parsley
- 1 tsp dried dill weed, crushed
- ¼ tsp oregano
- ¼ tsp coriander
- ¼ tsp ground cumin
- ¼ tsp salt
- 4 pita halves

Suggested Toppings:
- Red onion, slivered
- Seedless cucumber, thinly sliced
- Crumbled feta cheese
- Sliced black olives
- Chopped fresh peppers

Directions:
1. Stir dressing ingredients together and refrigerate while preparing lamb.
2. Combine all meatball ingredients in a large bowl and stir to distribute seasonings.
3. Shape the meat mixture into 12 small meatballs, rounded or slightly flattened if you prefer.
4. Air fry at 390°F (199°C) for 5 to 7 minutes, until well done. Remove and drain on paper towels.
5. To serve, pile meatballs and your choice of toppings in pita pockets and drizzle with dressing.

Nutrition:
- Calories: 270
- Fat: 14 g
- Protein: 18 g
- Carbs: 18 g
- Fiber: 2 g
- Sugar: 2 g
- Sodium: 618 mg

70. Rosemary Lamb Chops

Preparation Time: 30 minutes
Cooking Time: 20 minutes
Servings: 2 to 3
Ingredients:
- 2 tsp oil
- ½ tsp ground rosemary
- ½ tsp lemon juice
- 1 lb. (454 g) lamb chops, approximately 1-inch thick
- Salt and pepper, to taste

- Cooking spray

Directions:
1. Mix the oil, rosemary, and lemon juice, and rub into all sides of the lamb chops. Season to taste with salt and pepper.
2. For best flavor, cover lamb chops and allow them to rest in the fridge for 15 to 20 minutes.
3. Spray air fryer basket with nonstick spray and place lamb chops in it.
4. Air fry at 360°F (182°C) for approximately 20 minutes. This will cook chops to medium. The meat will be juicy but have no remaining pink. Air fry for 1 to 2 minutes longer for well-done chops. For rare chops, stop cooking after about 12 minutes and check for doneness.

Nutrition:
- Calories: 237
- Fat: 13 g
- Protein: 30 g
- Carbs: 0 g
- Fiber: 0 g
- Sugar 0 g
- Sodium: 116 mg

71. Delicious Meatballs

Preparation Time: 15 Minutes
Cooking Time: 25 Minutes
Servings: 6
Ingredients:
- 200 g ground beef
- 200 g ground chicken
- 100 g ground pork
- 30 g minced garlic
- 1 potato
- 1 egg
- 1 tsp basil
- 1 tsp cayenne pepper
- 1 tsp white pepper
- 2 tsp olive oil

Directions:
1. Combine ground beef, chicken meat, and pork in the mixing bowl, and stir it gently.
2. Sprinkle it with basil, cayenne pepper, and white pepper.
3. Add minced garlic and egg.
4. Stir the mixture gently. You should get a fluffy mass.
5. Peel the potato and grate it.
6. Add grated potato to the mixture and stir it again.
7. Preheat the air fryer oven to 180°C.
8. Take a tray and spray it with olive oil.

9. Make the balls from the meat mass and put them on the tray.
10. Lay the tray in the oven and cook it for 25 minutes.

Nutrition:
- Calories: 204
- Proteins: 26.0 g
- Fats: 7.6 g
- Carbohydrates: 7.1 g

72.   Low-fat Steak

Preparation Time: 25 Minutes
Cooking Time: 10 Minutes
Servings: 3

Ingredients:
- 400 g beef steak
- 1 tsp white pepper
- 1 tsp turmeric
- 1 tsp cilantro
- 1 tsp olive oil
- 3 tsp lemon juice
- 1 tsp oregano
- 1 tsp salt
- 100 ml water

Directions:
1. Rub the steaks with white pepper and turmeric, and put them in the big bowl.
2. Sprinkle the meat with salt, oregano, cilantro, and lemon juice.
3. Leave the steaks for 20 minutes.
4. Combine olive oil and water, and pour it into the bowl with steaks.
5. Grill the steaks in the air fryer for 10 minutes from both sides.
6. Serve it immediately.

Nutrition:
- Calories: 268
- Proteins: 40.7 g
- Fats: 10.1 g
- Carbohydrates: 1.4 g

73.   Diet Boiled Ribs

Preparation Time: 10 Minutes
Cooking Time: 30 Minutes
Servings: 4

Ingredients:
- 400 g pork ribs
- 1 tsp black pepper
- 1 g bay leaf
- 1 tsp basil
- 1 white onion
- 1 carrot
- 1 tsp cumin
- 700 ml water

Directions:
1. Cut the ribs on the portions and sprinkle them with black pepper.
2. Take a big saucepan and pour water into it.
3. Add the ribs and bay leaf.
4. Peel the onion and carrot, and add them to the water with the meat.
5. Sprinkle it with cumin and basil.
6. Cook it on medium heat in the air fryer for 30 minutes.

Nutrition:
- Calories: 294
- Proteins: 27.1 g
- Fats: 17.9 g
- Carbohydrates: 4.8 g

74.   Meatloaf

Preparation Time: 15 Minutes
Cooking Time: 30 Minutes
Servings: 4

Ingredients:
- 300 g ground beef
- 1 egg
- 1 onion
- 100 g carrot
- 1 tsp black pepper
- 1 tsp chili pepper
- 2 tsp olive oil

Directions:
1. Take the ground beef and put it in the big bowl.
2. Add egg, black pepper, and chili pepper. Stir the mixture very carefully.
3. Peel the carrot and onion, and chop it.
4. Add the chopped carrot and onion to the bowl with meat and stir it carefully.
5. Preheat the air fryer to 200°C.
6. Meanwhile, take the tray and spray it inside with olive oil. Make the loaf from the meat and put it on the tray.
7. Lay the tray in the oven and cook it for 30 minutes.

Nutrition:
- Calories: 198
- Proteins: 24.7 g
- Fats: 8.1 g
- Carbohydrates: 5.6 g

75.   Beef with Mushrooms

Preparation Time: 15 Minutes
Cooking Time: 40 Minutes
Servings: 4

Ingredients:

- 300 g beef
- 150 g mushrooms
- 1 onion
- 1 tsp olive oil
- 100 g vegetable broth
- 1 tsp basil
- 1 tsp chili
- 30 g tomato juice

Directions:

1. For this recipe, you should take a solid piece of beef. Take the beef and pierce the meat with a knife.
2. Rub it with olive oil, basil, chili, and lemon juice.
3. Chop the onion and mushrooms, and soak them with vegetable broth.
4. Cook the vegetables for 5 minutes.
5. Take a big tray and put the meat in it. Add vegetable broth to the tray too. It will make the meat juicy.
6. Preheat the air fryer oven to 180°C and cook it for 35 minutes.

Nutrition:

- Caloric: 175
- Proteins: 24.9 g
- Fats: 6.2 g
- Carbohydrates: 4.4 g

76.   Quick and Juicy Pork Chops

Preparation Time: 10 minutes
Cooking Time: 12 minutes
Servings: 4

Ingredients:

- 4 pork chops
- 1 tsp. olive oil
- 1 tsp. onion powder
- 1 tsp. paprika
- Pepper
- Salt

Directions:

1. Cover pork chops with olive oil and season with paprika, onion powder, pepper, and salt.
2. Place the dehydrating tray in a multi-level air fryer basket and place the basket in the instant pot.
3. Place pork chops on dehydrating tray.

4. Seal the pot with the air fryer lid, select air fry mode, and then set the temperature to 380°F and timer for 12 minutes. Turn pork chops halfway through.
5. Serve and enjoy.

Nutrition:

- Calories: 270
- Fat: 21.1 g
- Carbohydrates: 0.8 g
- Sugar: 0.3 g
- Protein: 18.1 g
- Cholesterol: 69 mg

77.   Delicious and Tender Pork Chops

Preparation Time: 10 minutes
Cooking Time: 12 minutes
Servings: 2

Ingredients:

- 2 pork chops
- 1 Tbsp olive oil
- ¼ tsp garlic powder
- ½ tsp onion powder
- 1 tsp ground mustard
- 1 ½ tsp pepper
- 1 Tbsp paprika
- 2 Tbsp brown sugar
- 1 ½ tsp salt

Directions:

1. In a minor container, mix garlic powder, onion powder, mustard, paprika, pepper, brown sugar, and salt.
2. Cover pork chops with olive oil and rub with spice mixture.
3. Place the dehydrating tray in a multi-level air fryer basket and place the basket in the instant pot.
4. Place pork chops on dehydrating tray.
5. Seal the pot with the air fryer lid, select air fry mode, and then set the temperature to 400°F and timer for 12 minutes. Turn pork chops halfway through.
6. Serve and enjoy.

Nutrition:

- Calories: 375
- Fat: 27.9 g
- Carbohydrates: 13.1 g
- Sugar: 9.5 g
- Protein: 19.2 g
- Cholesterol: 69 mg

78.   Perfect Pork Chops

Preparation Time: 10 minutes
Cooking Time: 15 minutes
Servings: 4
Ingredients:
- 4 pork chops
- Pepper
- Salt

Directions:
1. Season pork chops with pepper and salt.
2. Place the dehydrating tray in a multi-level air fryer basket and place the basket in the instant pot.
3. Place pork chops on dehydrating tray.
4. Seal the pot with the air fryer lid, select air fry mode, and then set the temperature to 400°F and timer for 15 minutes. Turn pork chops halfway through.
5. Serve and enjoy.

Nutrition:
- Calories: 256
- Fat: 19.9 g
- Carbohydrates: 0 g
- Sugar: 0 g
- Protein: 18 g
- Cholesterol: 69 mg

79.   Herb Butter Lamb Chops

Preparation Time: 10 minutes
Cooking Time: 5 minutes
Servings: 4
Ingredients:
- 4 lamb chops
- 1 tsp. rosemary, diced
- 1 Tbsp butter
- Pepper
- Salt

Directions:
1. Season lamb chops with pepper and salt.
2. Place the dehydrating tray in a multi-level air fryer basket and place the basket in the instant pot.
3. Place lamb chops on dehydrating tray.
4. Seal the pot with the air fryer lid, select air fry mode, and then set the temperature to 400°F and timer for 5 minutes.
5. Mix butter and rosemary, and spread on overcooked lamb chops.
6. Serve and enjoy.

Nutrition:
- Calories: 278
- Fat: 12.8 g
- Carbohydrates: 0.2 g
- Sugar: 0 g
- Protein: 38 g
- Cholesterol: 129 mg

80.   Za'atar Lamb Chops

Preparation Time: 10 minutes
Cooking Time: 10 minutes
Servings: 4
Ingredients:
- 4 lamb loin chops
- ½ Tbsp Za'atar
- 1 Tbsp fresh lemon juice
- 1 tsp. olive oil
- 2 garlic cloves, minced
- Pepper
- Salt

Directions:
1. Coat lamb chops with oil and lemon juice, and rub with Za'atar, garlic, pepper, and salt.
2. Place the dehydrating tray in a multi-level air fryer basket and place the basket in the instant pot.
3. Place lamb chops on dehydrating tray.
4. Seal the pot with the air fryer lid, select air fry mode, and then set the temperature to 400°F and timer for 10 minutes. Turn lamb chops halfway through.
5. Serve and enjoy.

Nutrition:
- Calories: 266
- Fat: 11.2 g
- Carbohydrates: 0.6 g
- Sugar: 0.1 g
- Protein: 38 g
- Cholesterol: 122 mg

Chapter 6.   Poultry Recipes

81.   Warm Chicken and Spinach Salad

Preparation Time: 10 Minutes
Cooking Time: 16 to 20 Minutes
Servings: 4
Ingredients:

- 3 (5 oz.) low-sodium boneless, skinless chicken breasts, cut into 1-inch cubes
- 5 tsp olive oil
- ½ tsp dried thyme
- 1 medium red onion, sliced
- 1 red bell pepper, sliced
- 1 small zucchini, cut into strips
- 3 Tbsp freshly squeezed lemon juice
- 6 cups fresh baby spinach

Directions:

1. In a huge bowl, blend the chicken with olive oil and thyme. Toss to coat. Transfer to a medium metal bowl and roast for 8 minutes in the air fryer.
2. Add the red onion, red bell pepper, and zucchini. Roast for 8 to 12 minutes more, stirring once during cooking, or until the chicken reaches an inner temperature of 165°F on a meat thermometer.
3. Remove the bowl from the air fryer and stir in the lemon juice.
4. Lay the spinach in a serving bowl and top with the chicken mixture. Toss to combine and serve immediately.

Nutrition:

- Calories: 214
- Fat: 7 g (29% of calories from fat)
- Saturated Fat: 1 g
- Protein: 28 g
- Carbohydrates: 7 g
- Sodium: 116 mg
- Fiber: 2 g
- Sugar 4 g
- 90% DV vitamin A
- 69% DV vitamin C

82.   Chicken in Tomato Juice

Preparation Time: 20 Minutes
Cooking Time: 15 Minutes
Servings: 3
Ingredients:

- 350 g chicken fillet

- 200 g tomato juice
- 100 g tomatoes
- 2 tsp basil
- 1 tsp chili
- 1 tsp oregano
- 1 tsp rosemary
- 1 tsp olive oil
- 1 tsp mint
- 1 tsp lemon juice

Directions:

1. Take a bowl and make the tomato sauce: combine basil, chili, oregano, rosemary, olive oil, mint, and lemon juice, and stir the mixture carefully.
2. You can use a hand mixer to mix the mass. It will make the mixture smooth.
3. Take a chicken fillet and separate it into three pieces.
4. Put the meat in the tomato mixture and leave for 15 minutes.
5. Meanwhile, preheat the air fryer oven to 230°C.
6. Put the meat mixture on the tray and put it in the oven for at least 15 minutes.

Nutrition:

- Calories: 258
- Proteins: 34.8 g
- Fats: 10.5 g
- Carbohydrates: 5.0 g

83.   Chicken Wings with Curry

Preparation Time: 15 Minutes
Cooking Time: 20 Minutes
Servings: 4
Ingredients:

- 400 g chicken wings
- 30 g curry
- 1 tsp chili
- 1 tsp cayenne pepper
- 1 tsp salt
- 1 lemon
- 1 tsp basil
- 1 tsp oregano
- 3 tsp mustard
- 1 tsp olive oil

Directions:

1. Rub the wings with chili, curry, cayenne pepper, salt, basil, and oregano.

2. Put it in a bowl and mix it carefully.
3. Leave the mixture at least for 10 minutes in the fridge.
4. Take away the mixture from the fridge and add mustard, and sprinkle with chopped lemon. Stir the mix gently again.
5. Sprig the pan with olive oil and put the wings in it.
6. Preheat the air fryer oven to 180°C and put wings there.
7. Cook it for 20 minutes.

Nutrition:

- Calories: 244
- Proteins: 30.8 g
- Fats: 10.6 g
- Carbohydrates: 7.2 g

84.   Chicken Meatballs

Preparation Time: 15 Minutes
Cooking Time: 20 Minutes
Servings: 6

Ingredients:

- 400 g ground chicken
- 100 g chopped dill
- 2 tsp olive oil
- 100 ml tomato juice
- 1 tsp black pepper
- 1 tsp white pepper
- 1 egg
- 20 ml milk

Directions:

1. Put the ground mix in a big mixing bowl.
2. Add chopped dill, black and white pepper, and stir the mixture carefully.
3. Add egg and stir it again.
4. Make the balls from the mixture and make the sauce from tomato juice and milk.
5. Pour the sauce into the tray and put the meatballs in it.
6. Preheat the air fryer oven to 180°C and put the meatballs in it.
7. Cook it for 20 minutes and serve immediately.

Nutrition:

- Calories: 199
- Proteins: 23.9 g
- Fats: 8.1 g
- Carbohydrates: 10.7 g

85.   Stuffed Chicken

Preparation Time: 15 Minutes
Cooking Time: 30 Minutes
Servings: 4

Ingredients:

- 2 chicken breasts
- 2 tomatoes
- 200 g basil
- 1 tsp black pepper
- 1 tsp cayenne pepper
- 100 ml tomato juice
- 40 g goat's cheese

Directions:

1. Make a "pocket" from chicken breasts and rub it with black pepper and cayenne pepper.
2. Slice tomatoes and chop basil.
3. Chop the goat cheese.
4. Combine all the ingredients — it will be the filling for breasts.
5. Fill the chicken breasts with this mixture.
6. Take a needle and thread and sew "pockets."
7. Preheat the air fryer oven to 200°C. Put the chicken breasts in the tray and pour it with tomato juice.
8. Serve.

Nutrition:

- Calories: 312
- Proteins: 41.6 g
- Fats: 13.4 g
- Carbohydrates: 5.6 g

86.   Duo Crisp Chicken Wings

Preparation Time: 10 minutes
Cooking Time: 18 minutes
Servings: 6

Ingredients:

- 12 chicken vignettes
- 1/2 cup chicken broth
- Salt and black pepper, to taste
- 1/4 cup melted butter

Directions:

1. Set a metal rack in the Instant Pot Duo Crisp and pour broth into it.
2. Place the vignettes on the metal rack, then put on its pressure-cooking lid.
3. Hit the "Pressure Button" and select 8 minutes of cooking time, then press "Start."
4. Once the Instant Pot Duo beeps, do a quick release and remove its lid.
5. Transfer the pressure-cooked vignettes to a plate.
6. Empty the pot and set an Air Fryer Basket in the Instant Pot Duo
7. Toss the vignettes with butter and seasoning.
8. Spread the seasoned vignettes in the Air Fryer Basket.

9. Put on the Air Fryer lid, hit the Air fryer Button, and then set the time to 10 minutes.
10. Remove the lid and serve.
11. Enjoy!

Nutrition:
- Calories: 246
- Total Fat: 18.9 g
- Saturated Fat: 7 g
- Cholesterol: 115 mg
- Sodium: 149 mg
- Total Carbohydrate: 0 g
- Dietary Fiber: 0 g
- Total Sugars: 0 g
- Protein: 20.2 g

87. Italian Whole Chicken

Preparation Time: 10 minutes
Cooking Time: 35 minutes
Servings: 4

Ingredients:
- 1 whole chicken
- 2 Tbsp or spray oil of choice
- 1 tsp garlic powder
- 1 tsp onion powder
- 1 tsp paprika
- 1 tsp Italian seasoning
- 2 Tbsp Montreal steak seasoning
- 1.5 cup chicken broth

Directions:
1. Whisk all the seasoning in a bowl and rub it on the chicken.
2. Set a metal rack in the Instant Pot Duo Crisp and pour broth into it.
3. Place the chicken on the metal rack, then put on its pressure-cooking lid.
4. Hit the "Pressure Button" and select 25 minutes of cooking time, then press "Start."
5. Once the Instant Pot Duo beeps, do a natural release and remove its lid.
6. Transfer the pressure-cooked chicken to a plate.
7. Empty the pot and set an Air Fryer Basket in the Instant Pot Duo.
8. Toss the chicken pieces with oil to coat well.
9. Spread the seasoned chicken in the air Fryer Basket.
10. Put on the Air Fryer lid, hit the Air fryer Button, and then set the time to 10 minutes.
11. Remove the lid and serve.
12. Enjoy!

Nutrition:
- Calories: 163

- Total Fat: 10.7 g
- Saturated Fat: 2 g
- Cholesterol: 33 mg
- Sodium: 1439 mg
- Total Carbohydrate: 1.8 g
- Dietary Fiber: 0.3 g
- Total Sugars: 0.8 g
- Protein: 12.6 g

88. Chicken Pot Pie

Preparation Time: 10 minutes
Cooking Time: 17 minutes
Servings: 6

Ingredients:
- 2 Tbsp olive oil
- 1 lb. chicken breast, cubed
- 1 Tbsp garlic powder
- 1 Tbsp thyme
- 1 Tbsp pepper
- 1 cup chicken broth
- 12 oz. bag frozen mixed vegetables
- 4 large potatoes cubed
- 10 oz. Can cream of chicken soup
- 1 cup heavy cream
- 1 pie crust
- 1 egg
- 1 Tbsp water

Directions:
1. Hit Sauté on the Instant Pot Duo Crispy and add the chicken and olive oil.
2. Sauté the chicken for 5 minutes, then stirs in spices.
3. Pour in the broth along with vegetables and cream of chicken soup
4. Put on the pressure-cooking lid and seal it.
5. Hit the "Pressure Button" and select 10 minutes of cooking time, then press "Start."
6. Once the Instant Pot Duo beeps, do a quick release and remove its lid.
7. Remove the lid and stir in cream.
8. Hit sauté and cook for 2 minutes.
9. Enjoy!

Nutrition:
- Calories: 568
- Total Fat: 31.1 g
- Saturated Fat: 9.1 g
- Cholesterol: 95 mg
- Sodium: 1111 mg
- Total Carbohydrate: 50.8 g
- Dietary Fiber: 3.9 g

- Total Sugars: 18.8 g
- Protein: 23.4 g

89.   Chicken Casserole

Preparation Time: 10 Minutes
Cooking Time: 9 minutes
Servings: 6
Ingredients:

- 3 cup chicken, shredded
- 12 oz. bag egg noodles
- ½ large onion
- ½ cup chopped carrots
- ¼ cup frozen peas
- ¼ cup frozen broccoli pieces
- 2 stalks celery chopped
- 5 cup chicken broth
- 1 tsp garlic powder
- Salt and pepper, to taste
- 1 cup cheddar cheese, shredded
- 1 package French's onions
- ¼ cup sour cream
- 1 can cream of chicken and mushroom soup

Directions:

1. Add chicken broth, black pepper, salt, garlic powder, vegetables, and egg noodles to the Instant Pot Duo.
2. Please put on the pressure-cooking lid and seal it.
3. Hit the "Pressure Button" and select 4 minutes of cooking time, then press "Start."
4. Once the Instant Pot Duo beeps, do a quick release and remove its lid.
5. Stir in cheese, 1/3 of French's onions, and the can of soup and sour cream.
6. Mix well and spread the remaining onion on top.
7. Could you put on the Air Fryer lid and seal it?
8. Hit the "Air fryer Button" and select 5 minutes of cooking time, then press "Start."
9. Once the Instant Pot Duo beeps, remove its lid.
10. Serve.

Nutrition:

- Calories: 494
- Total Fat: 19.1 g
- Saturated Fat: 9.6 g
- Cholesterol: 142 mg
- Sodium: 1233 mg
- Total Carbohydrate: 29 g
- Dietary Fiber: 2.6 g
- Total Sugars: 3.7 g
- Protein: 48.9 g

90.   Ranch Chicken Wings

Preparation Time: 10 minutes
Cooking Time: 35 minutes
Servings: 6
Ingredients:

- 12 chicken wings
- 1 Tbsp olive oil
- 1 cup chicken broth
- ¼ cup butter
- ½ cup Red Hot Sauce
- ¼ tsp Worcestershire sauce
- 1 Tbsp white vinegar
- ¼ tsp cayenne pepper
- 1/8 tsp garlic powder
- Seasoned salt, to taste
- Ranch dressing for dipping Celery, for garnish

Directions:

1. Set the Air Fryer Basket in the Instant Pot Duo and pour the broth into it.
2. Spread the chicken wings in the basket and put on the pressure-cooking lid.
3. Hit the "Pressure Button" and select 10 minutes of cooking time, then press "Start."
4. Meanwhile, for the sauce, add butter, vinegar, cayenne pepper, garlic powder, Worcestershire sauce, and spicy sauce in a small saucepan.
5. Stir and cook this sauce for 5 minutes on medium heat until it thickens.
6. Once the Instant Pot Duo beeps, do a quick release and remove its lid.
7. Remove the wings and empty the Instant Pot Duo.
8. Toss the wings with oil, salt, and black pepper.
9. Set the Air Fryer Basket in the Instant Pot Duo and arrange the wings into it.
10. Put on the Air Fryer lid and seal it.
11. Hit the "Air Fryer Button" and select 20 minutes of cooking time, then press "Start."
12. Once the Instant Pot Duo beeps, remove its lid.
13. Transfer the wings to the sauce and mix well.
14. Serve.

Nutrition:

- Calories: 414
- Total Fat: 31.6 g
- Saturated Fat: 11 g
- Cholesterol: 98 mg
- Sodium: 568 mg
- Total Carbohydrate: 11.2 g
- Dietary Fiber: 0.3 g
- Total Sugars: 0.2 g
- Protein: 20.4 g

91.   Chicken Mac and Cheese

Preparation Time: 10 minutes
Cooking Time: 9 minutes
Servings: 6

Ingredients:

- 2 ½ cup macaroni
- 2 cup chicken stock
- 1 cup cooked chicken, shredded
- 1 ¼ cup heavy cream
- 8 Tbsp butter
- 2 2/3 cups cheddar cheese, shredded
- 1/3 cup parmesan cheese, shredded
- 1 bag Ritz crackers
- ¼ tsp garlic powder
- Salt and pepper, to taste

Directions:

1. Add chicken stock, heavy cream, chicken, 4 Tbsp butter, and macaroni to the Instant Pot Duo.
2. Put on the pressure-cooking lid and seal it.
3. Hit the "Pressure Button" and select 4 minutes of cooking time, then press "Start."
4. Crush the crackers and mix them well with 4 Tbsp of melted butter.
5. Once the Instant Pot Duo beeps, do a quick release and remove its lid.
6. Put on the Air Fryer lid and seal it.
7. Hit the "Air Fryer Button" and select 5 minutes of cooking time, then press "Start."
8. Once the Instant Pot Duo beeps, remove its lid.
9. Serve.

Nutrition:

- Calories: 611
- Total Fat: 43.6 g
- Saturated Fat: 26.8 g
- Cholesterol: 147 mg
- Sodium: 739 mg
- Total Carbohydrate: 29.5 g
- Dietary Fiber: 1.2 g
- Total Sugars: 1.7 g
- Protein: 25.4 g

92.   Broccoli Chicken Casserole

Preparation Time: 10 minutes
Cooking Time: 22 minutes
Servings: 6

Ingredients:

- 1 ½ lb. chicken, cubed
- 2 tsp chopped garlic
- 2 Tbsp butter
- 1 ½ cups chicken broth
- 1 ½ cups long-grain rice
- 1 (10.75 oz.) can cream of chicken soup
- 2 cups broccoli florets
- 1 cup crushed Ritz cracker
- 2 Tbsp melted butter
- 2 cups shredded cheddar cheese

Directions:

1. Introduce 1 cup water to the Instant Pot Dup and place a basket in it.
2. Place the broccoli in the basket evenly.
3. Put on the pressure-cooking lid and seal it.
4. Hit the "Pressure Button" and select 1 minute of cooking time, then press "Start."
5. Once the Instant Pot Duo beeps, do a quick release and remove its lid.
6. Remove the broccoli and empty the Instant Pot Duo.
7. Hit the sauté button, then add 2 Tbsp of butter.
8. Toss in chicken, stir to cook for 5 minutes, and add garlic and sauté for 30 seconds.
9. Stir in rice, chicken broth, and cream of chicken soup.
10. Put on the pressure-cooking lid and seal it.
11. Hit the "Pressure Button" and select 12 minutes of cooking time, then press "Start."
12. Once the Instant Pot Duo beeps, do a quick release and remove its lid.
13. Add cheese and broccoli, then mix well gently.
14. Toss the cracker with 2 Tbsp of butter in a bowl and spread over the pot's chicken.
15. Could you put on the Air Fryer lid and seal it?
16. Hit the "Air Fryer Button" and select 4 minutes of cooking time, then press "Start."
17. Once the Instant Pot Duo beeps, remove its lid.
18. Serve.

Nutrition:

- Calories: 609
- Total Fat: 24.4 g
- Saturated Fat: 12.6 g
- Cholesterol: 142 mg
- Sodium: 924 mg
- Total Carbohydrate: 45.5 g
- Dietary Fiber: 1.4 g
- Total Sugars: 1.6 g
- Protein: 49.2 g

93.   Chicken Tikka Kebab

Preparation Time: 10 minutes
Cooking Time: 17 minutes
Servings: 4

Ingredients:

- 1 lb. chicken thighs boneless skinless, cubed

- 1 Tbsp oil
- ½ cup red onion, cubed
- ½ cup green bell pepper, cubed
- ½ cup red bell pepper, cubed
- Lime wedges to garnish
- Onion rounds to garnish

For marinade:

- ½ cup yogurt Greek
- ¾ Tbsp ginger, grated
- ¾ Tbsp garlic, minced
- 1 Tbsp lime juice
- 2 tsp red chili powder mild
- ½ tsp ground turmeric
- 1 tsp garam masala
- 1 tsp coriander powder
- ½ Tbsp dried fenugreek leaves
- 1 tsp salt

Directions:

1. Prepare the marinade by mixing yogurt with all its ingredients in a bowl.
2. Fold in chicken, then mix well to coat and refrigerate for 8 hours.
3. Add bell pepper, onions, and oil to the marinade, and mix well.
4. Yarn the chicken, peppers, and onions on the skewers.
5. Set the Air Fryer Basket in the Instant Pot Duo.
6. Put on the Air Fryer lid and seal it.
7. Hit the "Air Fry Button" and select 10 minutes of cooking time, then press "Start."
8. Once the Instant Pot Duo beeps, and remove its lid.
9. Flip the skewers and continue Air frying for 7 minutes.
10. Serve.

Nutrition:

- Calories: 241
- Total Fat: 14.2 g
- Saturated Fat: 3.8 g
- Cholesterol: 92 mg
- Sodium: 695 mg
- Total Carbohydrate: 8.5 g
- Dietary Fiber: 1.6 g
- Total Sugars: 3.9 g
- Protein: 21.8 g

94.   Bacon-Wrapped Chicken

Preparation Time: 10 minutes
Cooking Time: 24 minutes
Servings: 4

Ingredients:

- ¼ cup maple syrup
- 1 tsp ground black pepper
- 1 tsp Dijon mustard
- ¼ tsp garlic powder
- 1/8 tsp kosher salt
- 4 (6 oz.) skinless, boneless chicken breasts
- 8 slices bacon

Directions:

1. Whisk maple syrup with salt, garlic powder, mustard, and black pepper in a small bowl.
2. Rub the chicken with salt and black pepper and wrap each chicken breast with two slices of bacon.
3. Place the wrapped chicken in the Instant Pot baking pan.
4. Brush the wrapped chicken with maple syrup mixture.
5. Put on the Air Fryer lid and seal it.
6. Hit the "Bake Button" and select 20 minutes of cooking times, then press "Start."
7. Once the function is completed, switch the pot to Broil mode and broil for 4 minutes.
8. Serve.

Nutrition:

- Calories: 441
- Total Fat: 18.3 g
- Saturated Fat: 5.2 g
- Cholesterol: 141 mg
- Sodium: 1081 mg
- Total Carbohydrate: 14 g
- Dietary Fiber: 0.1 g
- Total Sugars: 11.8 g
- Protein: 53.6 g

95.   Creamy Chicken Thighs

Preparation Time: 10 minutes
Cooking Time: 25 minutes
Servings: 6

Ingredients:

- 1 Tbsp olive oil
- 6 chicken thighs, bone-in, skin-on
- Salt
- Freshly ground black pepper
- 2 cloves garlic, minced
- 1 Tbsp fresh thyme leaves
- 1 tsp crushed red pepper flakes
- 3/4 cup low-sodium chicken broth
- 1/2 cup heavy cream
- 1/2 cup sun-dried tomatoes, chopped
- 1/4 cup Parmesan, grated
- Freshly torn basil, for serving

Directions:

1. Hit sauté on the Instant Pot Duo Crisp and add oil to heat.
2. Stir in chicken, salt, and black, then sear for 5 minutes per side.
3. Add broth, cream, parmesan, and tomatoes.
4. Put on the Air Fryer lid and seal it.
5. Hit the "Bake Button" and select 20 minutes of cooking time, then press "Start."
6. Once the Instant Pot Duo beeps, remove its lid.
7. Garnish with basil and serve.

Nutrition:

- Calories: 454
- Total Fat: 37.8 g
- Saturated Fat: 14.4 g
- Cholesterol: 169 mg
- Sodium: 181 mg
- Total Carbohydrate: 2.8 g
- Dietary Fiber: 0.7 g
- Total Sugars: 0.7 g
- Protein: 26.9 g

96. Lemon Pepper Chicken

Preparation Time: 1 hour and 10 minutes
Cooking Time: 28 minutes
Servings: 4

Ingredients:

- 4 pastured chicken breasts
- ¼ cup lemon juice
- 3 Tbsps. Lemon-pepper seasoning
- 2 tips. Worcestershire sauce
- ¼ cup olive oil

Directions:

1. Prepare the marinade, and for this, place oil, Worcestershire sauce, salt, and lemon juice in a bowl, and whisk until combined.
2. Scratch each chicken breast into four pieces, add the chicken pieces into the marinade, toss until well coated, and marinate the chicken in the refrigerator for a minimum of 1 hour. Then, switch on the air fryer, insert the fryer basket, grease it with olive oil, then shut with its lid, set the fryer at 350°F, and preheat for 5 minutes.
3. Open the fryer, add chicken pieces in a single layer, spray with oil, close through its lid, and cook for 14 minutes at 350° F until nicely golden and cooked, turning the chicken halfway through the frying.
4. When the air fryer beeps, open its lid, transfer chicken onto a serving plate, and cook the remaining chicken pieces in the same manner. Serve hot.

Nutrition:

- Calories: 55
- Carbs: 1.3 g
- Fat: 2.7 g
- Protein: 6.6 g

97. Crumbed Poultry Tenderloins

Preparation Time: 15 minutes
Cooking Time: 12 minutes
Servings: 1

Ingredients:

- 1 egg
- ½ mug dry bread crumbs
- 2 Tbsp Vegetable oil
- 8 poultry tenderloins

Directions:

1. Adjust the air fryer temperature to 350°F.
2. Blend the egg in a small dish. Mix bread crumbs and oil in a second bowl until the mixture becomes loosened and crumbly.
3. Dip each poultry tenderloin into the egg dish; get rid of any residual egg. Dip tenderloins right into the crumb mix, making sure it is uniform and covered. Lay poultry tenderloins right into the basket of the air fryer. Prepare till no longer pink on the surface, about 12 mins. An instant-read thermometer inserted right into the center needs to review at least 165°F.

Nutrition:

- Calories: 253
- Carbs: 9.8 g
- Protein: 26.2
- Fat: 11.4 g

98. Air Fryer Barbeque Cheddar-Stuffed Poultry Breasts

Preparation Time: 10 minutes
Cooking Time: 25 minutes
Servings: 2

Ingredients:

- 3 divided strips bacon
- 2 oz. cubed cheddar cheese
- ¼ mug split BBQ sauce
- 4 oz. Skinless, boneless poultry breasts.
- Salt and black pepper

Directions:

1. Regulate the temperature of the air fryer to 380°F. Cook 1 strip of bacon in the air fryer for 2 mins. Remove from the air fryer and also cut into small

pieces. Line the air fryer and boost the temperature to 400°F.

2. Integrate cooked bacon, Cheddar cheese, and also 1 Tbsp. BBQ sauce in a bowl.

3. Utilize a long, sharp knife to make a horizontal 1-inch cut on top of each breast, producing a little interior bag. Stuff each bust with the bacon-cheese combination. Wrap continuing to place strips of bacon around each chicken bust. Coat the breast with remaining barbecue sauce and set it right into the ready air fryer basket.

4. Cook for 10 minutes in the air fryer, turn and proceed with food preparation till chicken is not pink in the center, and the juices run clear for 10 more minutes. An instant-read thermostat placed into the center needs to check out at the very least 165°F.

Nutrition:
- Calories: 379
- Carbs: 12.3 g
- Protein: 37.7 g
- Fat: 18.9 g

99. Air Fryer Hen Wings

Preparation Time: 5minutes
Cooking Time: 15 minutes
Servings: 4
Ingredients:
- 6 Chicken Wings — Flats and Drumettes
- Olive Oil Spray
- Salt
- Pepper
- Barbecue Sauce

Directions:
1. Splash the air fryer basket or foil-lined air fryer basket with non-stick cooking spray.
2. Arrange the wings equally into the basket. In a 4-quart air fryer basket, 6 wings fit well. Readjust this as required for the dimension of your air fryer.

3. Add an even layer of olive oil spray, a dashboard of salt and pepper to the wings.
4. Prepare at 390°F for 10 minutes.
5. Turn and also cook for an extra 10 minutes at 390°F.
6. Make sure the wings' internal temperature goes to the very least 165°F.
7. Coat with BBQ sauce if you prefer or other dipping sauces.

Nutrition:
- Calories: 308
- Protein: 17 g
- Fat: 11 g
- Carbs: 0 g

100. Air Fryer Teriyaki Hen Drumsticks

Preparation Time: 30 minutes
Cooking Time: 20 minutes
Servings: 4
Ingredients:
- 6 poultry drumsticks.
- 1 mug teriyaki sauce.
- Sesame seeds and onions, for garnish

Directions:
1. Mix drumsticks with teriyaki sauce in a zip lock bag. Allow sauce for half an hour.
2. Preheat air fryer to 361°F.
3. Place drumsticks in one layer in the air fryer basket and cook for 20 minutes. Shake the basket pair times through food preparation.
4. Garnish with sesame seeds as well as sliced environment-friendly onions

Nutrition:
- Calories: 163
- Carbs: 7 g
- Protein: 16 g
- Fat: 7 g

Chapter 7. Fish and Seafood Recipes

101. Mustard-Crusted Sole

Preparation Time: 5 Minutes
Cooking Time: 8 to 11 Minutes
Servings: 4

Ingredients:

- 5 tsp low-sodium yellow mustard
- 1 Tbsp freshly squeezed lemon juice
- 4 (3 ½ oz./99 g) sole fillets
- ½ tsp dried thyme
- ½ tsp dried marjoram
- 1/8 Tsp freshly ground black pepper
- 1 slice low-sodium whole-wheat bread, crumbled
- 2 tsp olive oil

Directions:

1. In a small bowl, blend the mustard and lemon juice. Spread this evenly over the fillets. Place them in the air fryer basket.
2. In another small bowl, mix the thyme, marjoram, pepper, bread crumbs, and olive oil. Mix until combined.
3. Gently but firmly, press the spice mixture onto each fish fillet's top.
4. Bake at 320°F (160°C) for 8 to 11 minutes, or until the fish reaches an inner temperature of at least 145°F (63°C) on a meat thermometer, and the topping is browned and crisp. Serve immediately.

Nutrition:

- Calories: 143
- Fat: 4 g
- Protein: 20 g
- Carbs: 5 g
- Fiber: 1 g
- Sugar 1 g
- Sodium: 140 mg

102. Almond Crusted Cod with Chips

Preparation Time: 10 Minutes
Cooking Time: 11 to 15 Minutes
Servings: 4

Ingredients:

- 2 russet potatoes, peeled, thinly sliced, rinsed, and patted dry
- 1 egg white
- 1 Tbsp freshly squeezed lemon juice
- 1/3 cup ground almonds
- 2 slices low-sodium whole-wheat bread, finely crumbled
- ½ tsp dried basil
- 4 (4 oz./113 g) cod fillets

Directions:

1. Preheat the oven to warm.
2. Put the potato slices in the air fryer basket and air fry at 390°F (199°C) for 11 to 15 minutes, or until crisp and brown. With tongs, turn the fries twice during cooking.
3. In the meantime, in a deep bowl, beat the egg white and lemon juice until frothy.
4. On a plate, mix the almonds, bread crumbs, and basil.
5. One at a time, dip the fillets into the egg white mixture and then into the almond-bread crumb mixture to coat. Place the coated fillets on a wire rack to dry while the fries cook.
6. When the potatoes are done, transfer them to a baking sheet and keep warm in the oven on low heat.
7. Air fry the fish in the air fryer basket for 10 to 14 minutes, or until the fish grasps an internal temperature of at least 140°F (60°C) on a meat thermometer and the coating is browned and crisp. Serve immediately with the potatoes.

Nutrition:

- Calories: 248
- Fat: 5 g
- Protein: 27 g
- Carbs: 25 g
- Fiber: 3 g
- Sugar 3 g
- Sodium: 131 mg

103. Honey Lemon Snapper with Fruit

Preparation Time: 15 Minutes
Cooking Time: 9 to 13 Minutes
Servings: 4

Ingredients:

- 4 (4 oz./113 g) red snapper fillets
- 2 tsp olive oil
- 3 nectarines, halved and pitted
- 3 plums, halved and pitted
- 1 cup red grapes
- 1 Tbsp freshly squeezed lemon juice
- 1 Tbsp honey

- ½ tsp dried thyme

Directions:
1. Put the red snapper in the air fryer basket and drizzle with the olive oil. Air fry at 390°F (199°C) for 4 minutes.
2. Remove the basket and add the nectarines and plums. Scatter the grapes overall.
3. Drizzle with the lemon juice and honey, and sprinkle with the thyme.
4. Transfer again the basket to the air fryer and air fry for 5 to 9 minutes more, or till the fish flakes, when tested with a fork, the fruit is tender. Serve immediately.

Nutrition:
- Calories: 246
- Fat: 4 g
- Protein: 25 g
- Carbs: 28 g
- Fiber: 3 g
- Sugar 24 g
- Sodium: 73 mg

104.   Easy Tuna Wraps

Preparation Time: 10 Minutes
Cooking Time: 4 to 7 Minutes
Servings: 4
Ingredients:
- 1 lb. (454 g) fresh tuna steak, cut into 1-inch cubes
- 1 Tbsp grated fresh ginger
- 2 garlic cloves, minced
- ½ tsp toasted sesame oil
- 4 low-sodium whole-wheat tortillas
- ¼ cup low-fat mayonnaise
- 2 cups shredded romaine lettuce
- 1 red bell pepper, thinly sliced

Directions:
1. In a medium bowl, mix the tuna, ginger, garlic, and sesame oil. Let it stand for 10 minutes, then transfer to the air fryer basket.
2. Air fry at 390°F (199°C) for 4 to 7 minutes, or until done to your liking and lightly browned.
3. Make wraps with tuna, tortillas, mayonnaise, lettuce, and bell pepper. Serve immediately.

Nutrition:
- Calories: 289
- Fat: 7 g
- Protein: 31 g
- Carbs: 26 g
- Fiber: 1 g
- Sugar 1 g
- Sodium: 135 mg

105.   Asian-Inspired Swordfish Steaks

Preparation Time: 10 Minutes
Cooking Time: 6 to 11 Minutes
Servings: 4
Ingredients:
- 4 (4 oz./113 g) swordfish steaks
- ½ tsp toasted sesame oil
- 1 jalapeño pepper, finely minced
- 2 garlic cloves, grated
- 1 Tbsp grated fresh ginger
- ½ tsp Chinese five-spice powder
- 1/8 Tsp freshly ground black pepper
- 2 Tbsp freshly squeezed lemon juice

Directions:
1. Place the swordfish steaks on a work surface and drizzle with the sesame oil.
2. In a small bowl, mix the jalapeño, garlic, ginger, five-spice powder, pepper, and lemon juice.
3. Rub this mixture into the fish and let it stand for 10 minutes.
4. Put in the air fryer basket.
5. Roast at 380°F (193°C) for 6 to 11 minutes, or until the swordfish reaches an inner temperature of at least 140°F (60°C) on a meat thermometer. Serve immediately.

Nutrition:
- Calories: 188
- Fat: 6 g
- Protein: 29 g
- Carbs: 2 g
- Fiber: 0 g
- Sugar: 1 g
- Sodium: 132 mg

106.   Salmon with Fennel and Carrot

Preparation Time: 15 Minutes
Cooking Time: 13 to 14 Minutes
Servings: 2
Ingredients:
- 1 fennel bulb, thinly sliced
- 1 large carrot, peeled and sliced
- 1 small onion, thinly sliced
- ¼ cup low-fat sour cream
- ¼ tsp coarsely ground pepper
- 2 (5 oz./142 g) salmon fillets

Directions:
1. Combine the fennel, carrot, and onion in a bowl, and toss.

2. Put the vegetable mixture into a baking pan. Cook in the air fryer at 400°F (204°C) for 4 minutes, or until the vegetables are crisp-tender.
3. Remove the pan from the air fryer. Stir in the sour cream and sprinkle the vegetables with pepper.
4. Top with the salmon fillets.
5. Return the pan to the air fryer. Roast for another 9 to 10 minutes, or until the salmon just barely flakes when tested with a fork.

Nutrition:
- Calories: 254
- Fat: 9 g
- Protein: 31 g
- Carbs: 12 g
- Fiber: 3 g
- Sugar 5 g
- Sodium: 115 mg

107.   Ranch Tilapia fillets

Preparation Time: 7 Minutes
Cooking Time: 17 Minutes
Servings: 2 fillets

Ingredients:
- 2 Tbsp flour
- 1 egg, lightly beaten
- 1 cup crushed cornflakes
- 2 Tbsp ranch seasoning
- 2 tilapia fillets
- Olive oil spray

Directions:
1. Place a parchment liner in the air fryer basket.
2. Scoop the flour out onto a plate; set it aside.
3. Put the beaten egg in a medium shallow bowl.
4. Introduce the cornflakes in a zip-top bag and crush them with a rolling pin or another small, blunt object.
5. On another plate, mix to combine the crushed cereal and ranch seasoning.
6. Dredge the tilapia fillets in the flour, dip in the egg, and press into the cornflake mixture.
7. Place the prepared fillets on the liner in the air fryer in a single layer.
8. Spray lightly with olive oil, and air fry at 400°F (204°C) for 8 minutes. Carefully flip the fillets and spray with more oil. Air fry for an additional 9 minutes, until golden and crispy, then serve.

Nutrition:
- Calories: 395
- Fat: 7 g
- Protein: 34 g
- Carbs: 49 g
- Fiber: 3 g

- Sugar 4 g
- Sodium: 980 mg

108.   Chilean Sea Bass with Green Olive Relish

Preparation Time: 10 Minutes
Cooking Time: 16 to 20 Minutes
Servings: 4

Ingredients:
- Olive oil spray
- 2 (6 oz./170 g) Chilean sea bass fillets or other firm-fleshed white fish
- 3 Tbsp extra-virgin olive oil
- ½ tsp ground cumin
- ½ tsp kosher salt
- ½ tsp black pepper
- 1/3 cup pitted green olives, diced
- ¼ cup finely diced onion
- 1 tsp chopped capers

Directions:
1. Spray the air fryer basket with olive oil spray. Drizzle the fillets with olive oil and sprinkle with cumin, salt, and pepper. Introduce the fish in the air fryer basket. Bake at 325°F (163°C) for 10 minutes or until the fish flakes easily with a fork.
2. In the meantime, in a small bowl, stir together the olives, onion, and capers.
3. Serve the fish topped with the relish.

Nutrition:
- Calories: 366
- Fat: 26 g
- Protein: 31 g
- Carbs: 2 g
- Fiber: 1 g
- Sugar: 0 g
- Sodium: 895 mg

109.   Ginger and Green Onion Fish

Preparation Time: 15 Minutes
Cooking Time: 15 Minutes
Servings: 2

Ingredients:
Bean Sauce:
- 2 Tbsp low-sodium soy sauce
- 1 Tbsp rice wine
- 1 Tbsp doubanjiang (Chinese black bean paste)
- 1 tsp minced fresh ginger
- 1 clove garlic, minced

Vegetables and Fish:
- 1 Tbsp peanut oil
- ¼ cup julienned green onions

- ¼ cup chopped fresh cilantro
- 2 Tbsp julienned fresh ginger
- 2 (6 oz./170 g) white fish fillets, such as tilapia

Directions:

For the sauce:
1. In a small bowl, combine all the ingredients and stir until well combined; set aside.

For the vegetables and fish:
1. In a medium bowl, combine the peanut oil, green onions, cilantro, and ginger. Toss to combine.
2. Cut two squares of parchment large enough to hold one fillet and half of the vegetables. Place one fillet on each parchment square, top with the vegetables, and pour over the sauce. Bend over the parchment paper and tuck the sides in small, tight folds to hold the fish, vegetables, and sauce securely inside the packet.
3. Place the packets in a single layer in the air fryer basket — roast at 350°F (177°C) for 15 minutes.
4. Transfer each packet to a dinner plate. Cut open with scissors just before serving.

Nutrition:
- Calories: 237
- Fat: 9 g
- Protein: 36 g
- Carbs: 3 g
- Fiber: 0 g
- Sugar: 0 g
- Sodium: 641 mg

110.   Asian Sesame Cod

Preparation Time: 5 Minutes
Cooking Time: 7 to 9 Minutes
Servings: 1

Ingredients:
- 1 Tbsp reduced-sodium soy sauce
- 2 tsp honey
- 1 tsp sesame seeds
- 6 oz. (170 g) cod fillet

Directions:
1. In a small bowl, combine the soy sauce and honey.
2. Cover the air fryer basket with nonstick cooking spray, then place the cod in the basket, brush with the soy mixture, and sprinkle sesame seeds on top. Roast at 360°F (182°C) for 7 to 9 minutes or until opaque.
3. Remove the fryer's fish and cool on a wire rack for 5 minutes before serving.

Nutrition:
- Calories: 141
- Fat: 1 g

- Protein: 26 g
- Carbs: 7 g
- Fiber: 1 g
- Sugar: 6 g
- Sodium: 466 mg

111.   Lemon Scallops with Asparagus

Preparation Time: 10 Minutes
Cooking Time: 7 to 10 Minutes
Servings: 4

Ingredients:
- ½ lb. (227 g) asparagus, ends trimmed and cut into 2-inch pieces
- 1 cup sugar snap peas
- 1 lb. (454 g) sea scallops
- 1 Tbsp lemon juice
- 2 tsp olive oil
- ½ tsp dried thyme
- Pinch salt
- Freshly ground black pepper, to taste

Directions:
1. Introduce the asparagus and sugar snap peas in the air fryer basket. Air fry at 400°F (204°C) for 2 to 3 minutes or until the vegetables are just getting tender.
2. Meanwhile, check the scallops for a small muscle attached to the side, and pull it off and discard.
3. In a medium bowl, toss the scallops with lemon juice, olive oil, thyme, salt, and pepper. Place into the air fryer basket on top of the vegetables.
4. Air fry for 5 to 7 minutes, tossing the basket once during the cooking time until the scallops are just firm when tested with your finger and are opaque in the center, and the vegetables are tender. Serve immediately.

Nutrition:
- Calories: 163
- Fat: 4 g
- Protein: 22 g
- Carbs: 10 g
- Fiber: 3 g
- Sugar: 3 g
- Sodium: 225 mg

112.   Fish Tacos

Preparation Time: 15 Minutes
Cooking Time: 9 to 12 Minutes
Servings: 4

Ingredients:
- 1 lb. (454 g) white fish fillets, such as snapper

- 1 Tbsp olive oil
- 3 Tbsp freshly squeezed lemon juice, divided
- 1½ cups chopped red cabbage
- ½ cup salsa
- 1/3 cup sour cream
- 6 whole-wheat tortillas
- 2 avocados, peeled and chopped

Directions:

1. Spray the fish with olive oil and sprinkle with 1 Tbsp of lemon juice. Place in the air fryer basket and air fry at 400°F (204°C) meant for 9 to 12 minutes or until the fish just flakes when tested with a fork.
2. Meanwhile, combine the remaining 2 Tbsp of lemon juice, cabbage, salsa, and sour cream in a medium bowl.
3. When the fish is cooked, remove it from the air fryer basket and break it into large pieces.
4. Let everyone assemble their taco combining the fish, tortillas, cabbage mixture, and avocados.

Nutrition:

- Calories: 547
- Fat: 27 g
- Protein: 33 g
- Carbs: 43 g
- Fiber: 12 g
- Sugar: 4 g
- Sodium: 679 mg

113.   Spicy Cajun Shrimp

Preparation Time: 7 Minutes
Cooking Time: 10 to 13 Minutes
Servings: 2 cups

Ingredients:

- ½ lb. (227 g) shrimp, peeled and deveined
- 1 Tbsp olive oil
- 1 tsp ground cayenne pepper
- ½ tsp Old Bay seasoning
- ½ tsp paprika
- 1/8 Tsp salt
- ½ a lemon, Juice

Directions:

1. In a huge bowl, syndicate the shrimp, olive oil, cayenne pepper, Old Bay Seasoning, paprika, and salt; toss to combine.
2. Transfer to the air fryer basket and roast at 390°F (199°C) for 10 to 13 minutes, until browned.
3. Sprinkle a bit of lemon juice over the shrimp before serving.

Nutrition:

- Calories: 159

- Fat: 7 g
- Protein: 23 g
- Carbs: 1 g
- Fiber: 0 g
- Sugar: 0 g
- Sodium: 291 mg

114.   Garlic Parmesan Roasted Shrimp

Preparation Time: 7 Minutes
Cooking Time: 10 to 13 Minutes
Servings: 4 cups

Ingredients:

- 1 lb. (454 g) jumbo shrimp, peeled and deveined
- 1/3 cup Parmesan cheese
- 1 Tbsp olive oil
- 1 tsp onion powder
- 2 tsp minced garlic
- ½ tsp ground black pepper
- ¼ tsp dried basil

Directions:

1. In a large bowl, toss to combine the shrimp, Parmesan cheese, olive oil, onion powder, garlic, pepper, and basil.
2. Transfer to the air fryer basket and roast at 350°F (177°C) for 10 to 13 minutes, until the shrimp are browned, and serve.

Nutrition:

- Calories: 162
- Fat: 6 g
- Protein: 25 g
- Carbs: 2 g
- Fiber: 0 g
- Sugar: 0 g
- Sodium: 271 mg

115.   Quick Shrimp Scampi

Preparation Time: 10 Minutes
Cooking Time: 7 to 8 Minutes
Servings: 2

Ingredients:

- 30 (1 lb./454 g) uncooked large shrimp, peeled, deveined, and tails removed
- 2 tsp olive oil
- 1 garlic clove, thinly sliced
- ½ lemon, Juice, and zest
- 1/8 Tsp kosher salt
- Pinch red pepper flakes (optional)
- 1 Tbsp chopped fresh parsley

Directions:

1. Sprig a baking pan with nonstick cooking spray, then combine the shrimp, olive oil, sliced garlic, lemon juice and zest, kosher salt, and red pepper flakes (if using) in the pan, tossing to coat—place in the air fryer basket.
2. Roast at 360°F (182°C) for 7 to 8 minutes or until firm and bright pink.
3. Remove the fish from the fryer, place it on a serving plate, and sprinkle the parsley on top. Serve warm.

Nutrition:

- Calories: 321
- Fat: 13 g
- Protein: 46 g
- Carbs: 5 g
- Fiber: 0 g
- Sugar: 1 g
- Sodium: 383 mg

116.   Mustard-Crusted Fish Fillets

Preparation Time: 5 Minutes
Cooking Time: 8 to 11 Minutes
Servings: 4

Ingredients:

- 5 tsp low-sodium yellow mustard (see Tip)
- 1 Tbsp freshly squeezed lemon juice
- 4 (3.5 oz.) sole fillets
- ½ tsp dried thyme
- ½ tsp dried marjoram
- 1/8 Tsp freshly ground black pepper
- 1 slice low-sodium whole-wheat bread, crumbled
- 2 tsp olive oil

Directions:

1. In a small bowl, stir the mustard and lemon juice. Spread this evenly over the fillets. Place them in the air fryer basket.
2. In another small bowl, mix the thyme, marjoram, pepper, bread crumbs, and olive oil. Mix until combined.
3. Gently but firmly, press the spice mixture onto each fish fillet's top.
4. Bake for 8 to 11 minutes, or until the fish reaches an internal temperature of at least 145°F on a meat thermometer and the topping is browned and crisp. Serve immediately.

Nutrition:

- Calories: 142
- Fat: 4 g (25% of calories from fat)
- Saturated Fat: 1 g
- Protein: 20 g

- Carbohydrates: 5 g
- Sodium: 140 g
- Fiber: 1 g
- Sugar: 1 g;
- 4 DV vitamin C

117.   Fish and Vegetable Tacos

Preparation Time: 15Minutes
Cooking Time: 9 to 12 Minutes
Servings: 4

Ingredients:

- 1 lb. white fish fillets, such as sole or cod
- 2 tsp olive oil
- 3 Tbsp freshly squeezed lemon juice, divided
- 1 ½ cups chopped red cabbage
- 1 large carrot, grated
- ½ cup low-sodium salsa
- 1/3 Cup low-fat Greek yogurt
- 4 soft low-sodium whole-wheat tortillas

Directions:

1. Scrub the fish with olive oil and drizzle with 1 Tbsp of lemon juice. Fry in the air fryer basket for 9 to 12 minutes, or till the fish just flakes when tested with a fork.
2. In the meantime, in a medium bowl, stir together the remaining 2 Tbsp of lemon juice, the red cabbage, carrot, salsa, and yogurt.
3. When the fish is cooked, remove it from the air fryer basket and break it up into large pieces.

Nutrition:

- Calories: 209
- Fat: 3 g (13% of calories from fat)
- Saturated Fat: 0 g
- Protein: 18 g
- Carbohydrates: 30 g
- Sodium: 116 mg
- Fiber: 1 g
- Sugar: 4 g
- 70% DV vitamin A
- 43% DV vitamin C

118.   Lighter Fish and Chips

Preparation Time: 10 Minutes
Cooking Time: 11 to 15 Minutes (Chips), 11 to 15 Minutes (Cod Fillets)
Servings: 4

Ingredients:

- 2 russet potatoes, peeled, thinly sliced, rinsed, and patted dry (see Tip)
- 1 egg white

- 1 Tbsp freshly squeezed lemon juice
- 1/3 cup ground almonds
- 2 slices low-sodium whole-wheat bread, finely crumbled
- ½ tsp dried basil
- 4 (4-oz.) cod fillets

Directions:

1. Preheat the oven to warm.
2. Put the potato slices in the air fryer basket and air-fry for 11 to 15 minutes, or until crisp and brown. With tongs, turn the fries twice during cooking.
3. In the meantime, in a shallow bowl, beat the egg white and lemon juice until frothy.
4. On a plate, mix the almonds, bread crumbs, and basil.
5. Separately, dip the fillets into the egg white mixture and then into the almond–bread crumb mixture to coat. Place the coated fillets on a wire rack to dry while the fries cook.
6. When the potatoes are done, transfer them to a baking sheet and keep warm in the oven on low heat
7. Air-fry the fish in the air fryer basket for 10 to 14 minutes, or until the fish grasps an inner temperature of at least 140°F on a meat thermometer and the coating is browned and crisp. Serve immediately with the potatoes.

Nutrition:

- Calories: 247
- Fat: 5 g (18% of calories from fat)
- Saturated Fat: 0 g
- Protein: 27 g
- Carbohydrates: 25 g
- Sodium: 131 mg
- Fiber: 3 g
- Sugar: 3 g
- 23% DV vitamin C

119. Snapper with Fruit

Preparation Time: 15 Minutes
Cooking Time: 9 to 13 Minutes
Servings: 4

Ingredients:

- 4 (4 oz.) red snapper fillets
- 2 tsp olive oil
- 3 nectarines, halved and pitted
- 3 plums, halved and pitted
- 1 cup red grapes
- 1 Tbsp freshly squeezed lemon juice
- 1 Tbsp honey
- ½ tsp dried thyme

Directions:

1. Put the red snapper in the air fryer basket and drizzle with the olive oil. Air-fry for 4 minutes.
2. Remove the basket and add the nectarines and plums. Scatter the grapes overall.
3. Drizzle with the lemon juice and honey, and sprinkle with the thyme.
4. Put back the basket to the air fryer and air-fry for 5 to 9 minutes more, or till the fish flakes, when tested with a fork, the fruit is tender. Serve immediately.

Nutrition:

- Calories: 245
- Fat: 4 g (15% of calories from fat)
- Saturated Fat: 1 g
- Protein: 25 g
- Carbohydrates: 28 g
- Sodium: 73 mg
- Fiber: 3 g
- Sugar: 24 g
- 11% DV vitamin A
- 27% DV vitamin C

120. Tuna and Fruit Kebabs

Preparation Time: 15 Minutes
Cooking Time: 8 to 12 Minutes
Servings: 4

Ingredients:

- 1 lb. tuna steaks, cut into 1-inch cubes
- ½ cup canned pineapple chunks, drained, juice reserved
- ½ cup large red grapes
- 1 Tbsp honey
- 2 tsp grated fresh ginger
- 1 tsp olive oil
- Pinch cayenne pepper

Directions:

1. Thread the tuna, pineapple, and grapes on 8 bamboos or 4 metal skewers that fit in the air fryer.
2. In a small bowl, whisk the honey, 1 Tbsp of reserved pineapple juice, ginger, olive oil, and cayenne. Brush this mixture over the kebabs. Let them stand for 10 minutes.
3. Grill the kebabs for 8 to 12 minutes, or until the tuna reaches an internal temperature of at least 145°F on a meat thermometer, and the fruit is tender and glazed, brushing once with the remaining sauce. Discard any remaining marinade. Serve immediately.

Nutrition:

- Calories: 181
- Fat: 2 g (10% of calories from fat)
- Saturated Fat: 0 g
- Protein: 18 g
- Carbohydrates: 13 g
- Sodium: 43 mg
- Fiber: 1 g
- Sugar: 12 g
- 3% DV vitamin A
- 6% DV vitamin C

Chapter 8.   Desserts Recipes

121.   Sweet Tapioca Pudding

Preparation Time: 10 minutes
Cooking Time: 8 minutes
Servings: 4
Ingredients:

- ½ cup pearl tapioca
- 1 can coconut milk
- ½ cup water
- 4 Tbsp maple syrup
- 1 cup almond milk
- Pinch cardamom

Directions:

1. Soak tapioca in almond milk for 1 hour.
2. Combine all ingredients except water into the heat-safe bowl and cover the bowl with foil.
3. Pour ½ cup water into the instant pot, then place trivet into the pot.
4. Place bowl on top of the trivet.
5. Cover the pot with the lid and cook on manual high pressure for 8 minutes.
6. Once done, allow to release pressure naturally, then open the lid.
7. Stir well — place in the refrigerator for 1 hour.
8. Serve and enjoy.

Nutrition:

- Calories: 313
- Fat: 18.1 g
- Carbohydrates: 38.4 g
- Sugar: 18.5 g
- Protein: 2.4 g
- Cholesterol: 1 mg

122.   Vanilla Bread Pudding

Preparation Time: 10 minutes
Cooking Time: 15 minutes
Servings: 4
Ingredients:

- 3 eggs, lightly beaten
- 1 tsp. coconut oil
- 1 tsp. vanilla
- 4 cup bread cube
- ½ tsp. cinnamon
- ¼ cup raisins
- ¼ cup chocolate chips
- 2 cup milk
- ¼ tsp. salt

Directions:

1. Add water into the instant pot, then place the trivet into the pot.
2. Add bread cubes to a baking dish.
3. In a large bowl, mix the remaining ingredients.
4. Pour the bowl mixture into the baking dish on top of bread cubes and cover the dish with foil.
5. Place baking dish on top of the trivet.
6. Seal the pot with the lid and cook on steam mode for 15 minutes.
7. Once done, allow to release pressure naturally, then open the lid.
8. Carefully remove the baking dish from the pot.
9. Serve and enjoy.

Nutrition:

- Calories: 230
- Fat:10.1 g
- Carbohydrates: 25 g
- Sugar: 16.7 g
- Protein: 9.2 g
- Cholesterol: 135 mg

123.   Blueberry Cupcakes

Preparation Time: 10 minutes
Cooking Time: 25 minutes
Servings: 6
Ingredients:

- 2 eggs, lightly beaten
- ¼ cup butter, softened
- ½ tsp. baking soda
- 1 tsp. baking powder
- 1 tsp. vanilla extract
- ½ fresh lemon juice
- 1 lemon zest
- ¼ cup sour cream
- ¼ cup milk
- 1 cup sugar
- ¾ cup fresh blueberries
- 1 cup all-purpose flour
- ¼ tsp. salt

Directions:

1. Add all ingredients into the large bowl and mix well.
2. Empty 1 cup of water into the instant pot, then place trivet into the pot.
3. Pour batter into the silicone cupcake mound and place it on top of the trivet.

4. Seal the pot with the lid and cook on manual high pressure for 25 minutes.
5. Once done, allow to release pressure naturally, then open the lid.
6. Serve and enjoy.

Nutrition:
- Calories: 330
- Fat: 11.6 g
- Carbohydrates: 53.6 g
- Sugar: 36 g
- Protein: 4.9 g
- Cholesterol: 80 mg

124. Moist Pumpkin Brownie

Preparation Time: 10 minutes
Cooking Time: 35 minutes
Servings: 4
Ingredients:
- 2 eggs, lightly beaten
- ¾ cup pumpkin puree
- ½ tsp. baking powder
- 1/3 cup cocoa powder
- ½ cup almond flour
- 1 Tbsp vanilla
- ¼ cup milk
- 1 cup maple syrup

Directions:
1. Place all ingredients into a large bowl and mix until well combined.
2. Spray spring-form pan with cooking spray.
3. Pour batter into the pan and cover the pan with foil.
4. Pour 2 cups of water into the instant pot and place trivet into the pot.
5. Put the cake pan on top of the trivet.
6. Close the pot with the lid and cook on manual mode for 35 minutes.
7. Once done, release pressure using the quick-release method, then open the lid.
8. Slice and serve.

Nutrition:
- Calories: 306
- Fat: 5.5 g
- Carbohydrates: 62.9 g
- Sugar: 49.9 g
- Protein: 5.8 g
- Cholesterol: 83 mg

125. Mini Choco Cake

Preparation Time: 10 minutes
Cooking Time: 9 minutes
Servings: 2
Ingredients:
- 2 eggs
- 2 Tbsp swerve
- ¼ cup cocoa powder
- ½ tsp vanilla
- ½ tsp baking powder
- 2 Tbsp heavy cream

Directions:
1. In a container, blend all dry ingredients until combined.
2. Add all wet ingredients to the dry mixture and whisk until smooth.
3. Spray 2 ramekins with cooking spray.
4. Introduce 1 cup of water into the instant pot, then place the trivet in the pot.
5. Pour batter into the ramekins and place ramekins on top of the trivet.
6. Close the pot with a lid and cook on manual high pressure for 9 minutes.
7. Once done, release pressure using the quick-release method, then open the lid.
8. Carefully remove ramekins from the pot and let it cool.
9. Serve and enjoy.

Nutrition:
- Calories: 143
- Fat: 11.3 g
- Carbohydrates: 22.4 g
- Sugar: 15.7 g
- Protein: 7.8 g
- Cholesterol: 184 mg

126. Cinnamon Pears

Preparation Time: 10 minutes
Cooking Time: 7 minutes
Servings: 4
Ingredients:
- 4 firm pears, peel
- ½ tsp nutmeg
- 1/3 cup sugar
- 1 tsp ginger
- 1 ½ tsp cinnamon
- 1 cinnamon stick
- 1 cup orange juice

Directions:

1. Add orange juice and all spices into the instant pot.
2. Place the trivet into the pot.
3. Arrange pears on top of the trivet.
4. Close the pot with a lid and cook on manual high pressure for 7 minutes.
5. Once done, allow to release pressure naturally, then open the lid.
6. Carefully remove pears from the pot and set them aside.
7. Discard cinnamon sticks and cloves from the pot.
8. Add sugar to the pot and set the pot on sauté mode.
9. Cook the sauce until thickened.
10. Pour the sauce over pears and serve.

Nutrition:

- Calories: 221
- Fat: 0.6 g
- Carbohydrates: 57.5 g
- Sugar: 42.4 g
- Protein: 1.3 g
- Cholesterol: 0 mg

127.   Delicious Pumpkin Pudding

Preparation Time: 10 minutes
Cooking Time: 20 minutes
Servings: 6

Ingredients:

- 2 large eggs, lightly beaten
- ½ cup milk
- ½ tsp vanilla
- 1 tsp pumpkin pie spice
- 14 oz. pumpkin puree
- ¾ cup swerve

Directions:

1. Lard a baking dish with cooking spray and set it aside.
2. In a large bowl, whisk eggs with the remaining ingredients.
3. Empty 1 ½ cups of water into the instant pot, then place a steamer rack in the pot.
4. Pour the mixture into the prepared dish and cover with foil.
5. Place dish on top of steamer rack.
6. Close the pot with a lid and cook on manual high pressure for 20 minutes.
7. As soon as done, discharge pressure naturally for 10 minutes and then release it using the quick-release method. Open the lid.
8. Carefully remove the dish from the pot and let it cool.
9. Place pudding dish in the refrigerator for 7–8 hours.

10. Serve and enjoy.

Nutrition:

- Calories: 58
- Fat: 2.3 g
- Carbohydrates: 36.7 g
- Sugar: 33.3 g
- Protein: 3.5 g
- Cholesterol: 64 mg

128.   Saffron Rice Pudding

Preparation Time: 10 minutes
Cooking Time: 10 minutes
Servings: 6

Ingredients:

- ½ cup rice
- ½ tsp cardamom powder
- 3 Tbsp almonds, chopped
- 3 Tbsp walnuts, chopped
- 4 cups milk
- ½ cup sugar
- 2 Tbsp shredded coconut
- 1 tsp saffron
- 3 Tbsp raisins
- 1 Tbsp ghee
- 1/8 tsp salt
- ½ Water

Directions:

1. Add ghee into the pot and set the pot on sauté mode.
2. Add rice and cook for 30 seconds.
3. Add 3 cups milk, coconut, raisins, saffron, nuts, cardamom powder, sugar, ½ cup water, and salt, and blending well.
4. Close the pot with a lid and cook on manual high pressure for 10 minutes.
5. Once done, release pressure naturally for 15 minutes and then release it using the quick-release method. Open the lid.
6. Add remaining milk and stir well; cook on sauté mode for 2 minutes.
7. Serve and enjoy.

Nutrition:

- Calories: 280
- Fat: 9.9 g
- Carbohydrates: 42.1 g
- Sugar: 27 g
- Protein: 8.2 g
- Cholesterol: 19 mg

129.   Flavorful Carrot Halva

Preparation Time: 10 minutes
Cooking Time: 10 minutes
Servings: 6
Ingredients:

- 2 cups carrots, shredded
- 2 Tbsp ghee
- ½ tsp cardamom
- 3 Tbsp ground cashews
- ¼ cup sugar
- 1 cup milk
- 4 Tbsp raw cashews
- 3 Tbsp raisins

Directions:

1. Add ghee to the instant pot and set the pot on sauté mode.
2. Add raisins and cashews, cook until lightly golden brown.
3. Add the remaining ingredients except for cardamom, blending well.
4. Close the pot with a lid and cook on manual high pressure for 10 minutes.
5. Once done, allow to release pressure naturally, then open the lid.
6. Add cardamom and stir well, serve.

Nutrition:

- Calories: 171
- Fat: 9.3 g
- Carbohydrates: 20.5 g
- Sugar: 15.2 g
- Protein: 3.3 g
- Cholesterol: 14 mg

130.   Vermicelli Pudding

Preparation Time: 10 minutes
Cooking Time: 2 minutes
Servings: 6
Ingredients:

- 1/3 cup vermicelli, roasted
- 6 dates, pitted, sliced
- 3 Tbsp cashews, slice
- 2 Tbsp pistachios, slice
- ¼ tsp vanilla
- ½ tsp saffron
- 1/3 cup sugar
- 5 cups milk
- 3 Tbsp shredded coconut
- 2 Tbsp raisins
- 3 Tbsp almonds
- 2 Tbsp ghee

Directions:

1. Add ghee to the instant pot and set the pot on sauté mode.
2. Add dates, cashews, pistachios, and almonds into the pot, and cook for a minute.
3. Add raisins, coconut, and vermicelli. Stir well.
4. Add 3 cups milk, saffron, and sugar. Blend well.
5. Close the pot with a lid and cook on manual high pressure for 2 minutes.
6. Once done, allow to release pressure naturally, then open the lid.
7. Stir remaining milk and vanilla.
8. Serve and enjoy.

Nutrition:

- Calories: 283
- Fat: 13.4 g
- Carbohydrates: 34.9 g
- Sugar: 28.1 g
- Protein: 9 g
- Cholesterol: 28 mg

131.   Yogurt Custard

Preparation Time: 10 minutes
Cooking Time: 20 minutes
Servings: 6
Ingredients:

- 1 cup plain yogurt
- 1 ½ tsp ground cardamom
- 1 cup sweetened condensed milk
- 1 cup milk

Directions:

1. Add all ingredients into the heat-safe bowl and stir to combine.
2. Cover the bowl with foil.
3. Pour 2 cups of water into the instant pot, then place the trivet in the pot.
4. Place the bowl on top of the trivet.
5. Close the pot with a lid and cook on manual high pressure for 20 minutes.
6. Once done, release pressure naturally for 20 minutes and then release it using the quick-release method. Open the lid.
7. Once the custard bowl is cool, place it in the refrigerator for 1 hour.
8. Serve and enjoy.

Nutrition:

- Calories: 215
- Fat: 5.8 g
- Carbohydrates: 33 g
- Sugar: 32.4 g
- Protein: 7.7 g
- Cholesterol: 23 mg

132.   Simple Raspberry Mug Cake

Preparation Time: 10 minutes
Cooking Time: 10 minutes
Servings: 3

Ingredients:

- 3 eggs
- 1 cup almond flour
- ½ tsp vanilla
- 1 Tbsp swerve
- 2 Tbsp chocolate chips
- ½ cup raspberries
- Pinch salt

Directions:

1. Add all ingredients into a large bowl and mix until well combined.
2. Pour 2 cups of water into the instant pot, then place a trivet in the pot.
3. Pour batter into the heat-safe mugs. Cover with foil and place on top of the trivet.
4. Close the pot with a lid and cook on manual high pressure for 10 minutes.
5. Once done, release pressure using the quick-release method, then open the lid.
6. Serve and enjoy.

Nutrition:

- Calories: 326
- Fat: 25.3 g
- Carbohydrates: 20 g
- Sugar: 11.3 g
- Protein: 11.3 g
- Cholesterol: 165 mg

133.   Chocolate Mousse

Preparation Time: 10 minutes
Cooking Time: 6 minutes
Servings: 5

Ingredients:

- 4 egg yolks
- ¼ cup water
- ½ cup sugar
- 1 tsp vanilla
- 1 cup heavy cream
- ½ cup cocoa powder
- ½ cup milk
- ¼ tsp sea salt

Directions:

1. Whisk egg yolks in a bowl until combined.
2. In a saucepan, add cocoa, water, and sugar, and whisk over medium heat until sugar is melted.

3. Add milk and cream to the saucepan and whisk to combine. Do not boil.
4. Add vanilla and salt; stir well.
5. Introduce 1 ½ cups water into the instant pot, then place a trivet in the pot.
6. Pour mixture into the ramekins and place on top of the trivet.
7. Close the pot with a lid and cook on manual mode for 6 minutes.
8. Once done, release pressure using the quick-release method, then open the lid.
9. Serve and enjoy.

Nutrition:

- Calories: 235
- Fat: 14.1 g
- Carbohydrates: 27.2 g
- Sugar: 21.5 g
- Protein: 5 g
- Cholesterol: 203 mg

134.   Cardamom Zucchini Pudding

Preparation Time: 10 minutes
Cooking Time: 10 minutes
Servings: 4

Ingredients:

- 1 ¾ cups zucchini, shredded
- 5 oz. half and half
- 5.5 oz. milk
- 1 tsp. cardamom powder
- 1/3 cup sugar

Directions:

1. Add all ingredients except cardamom into the instant pot and blend well.
2. Close the pot with a lid and cook on manual high pressure for 10 minutes.
3. As soon as done, discharge pressure naturally for 10 minutes and then release it using the quick-release method. Open the lid.
4. Stir in cardamom and serve.

Nutrition:

- Calories: 138
- Fat: 5 g
- Carbohydrates: 22.1 g
- Sugar: 19.4 g
- Protein: 3 g
- Cholesterol: 16 mg

135. Yummy Strawberry Cobbler

Preparation Time: 10 minutes
Cooking Time: 12 minutes
Servings: 3
Ingredients:

- 1 cup strawberries, sliced
- ½ tsp vanilla
- 1/3 cup butter
- 1 cup milk
- 1 tsp baking powder
- ½ cup granulated sugar
- 1 ¼ cup all-purpose flour

Directions:

1. In a huge container, add all ingredients except strawberries and stir to combine.
2. Add sliced strawberries and fold well.
3. Grease ramekins with cooking spray, then pour batter into the ramekins.
4. Discharge 1 ½ cups water into the instant pot, then place the trivet in the pot.
5. Place ramekins on top of the trivet.
6. Close the pot with a lid and cook on manual high pressure for 12 minutes.
7. As soon as done, discharge pressure naturally for 10 minutes and then release it using the quick-release method. Open the lid.
8. Serve and enjoy.

Nutrition:

- Calories: 555
- Fat: 22.8 g
- Carbohydrates: 81.7 g
- Sugar: 39.6 g
- Protein: 8.6 g
- Cholesterol: 61 mg

136. Peach Cobbler

Preparation Time: 10 minutes
Cooking Time: 20 minutes
Servings: 6
Ingredients:

- 20 oz. can peach pie filling
- 1 ½ tsp cinnamon
- ¼ tsp nutmeg
- 14.5 oz. vanilla cake mix
- ½ cup butter, melted

Directions:

1. Add peach pie filling into the instant pot.
2. In a bulky container, mix the remaining ingredients and spread them over peach pie filling.

3. Close the pot with a lid and cook on manual high pressure for 10 minutes.
4. As soon as done, discharge pressure naturally for 10 minutes and then release it using the quick-release method. Open the lid.
5. Serve and enjoy.

Nutrition:

- Calories: 445
- Fat: 15.4 g
- Carbohydrates: 76.1 g
- Sugar: 47.7 g
- Protein: 0.2 g
- Cholesterol: 41 mg

137. Hazelnuts Brownies

Preparation Time: 10 minutes
Cooking Time: 25 minutes
Servings: 6
Ingredients:

- 4 eggs
- 1 cup almond flour
- 4 Tbsp hazelnuts, chopped
- ¼ cup swerve
- ¼ cup cocoa powder
- 2 Tbsp butter
- ½ tsp vanilla
- ½ cup mascarpone
- ½ cup flaxseed meal

Directions:

1. In a huge bowl, swell all ingredients and beat until well combined.
2. Spray a baking dish with cooking spray.
3. Introduce 1 cup of water into the instant pot, then place a trivet in the pot.
4. Pour batter into the baking dish and place the dish on top of the trivet.
5. Close the pot with the lid and cook on manual high pressure for 25 minutes.
6. Once done, release pressure using the quick-release method, then open the lid.
7. Slice and serve.

Nutrition:

- Calories: 289
- Fat: 23.6 g
- Carbohydrates: 18.1 g
- Sugar: 11.3 g
- Protein: 12.3 g
- Cholesterol: 130 mg

138.   Apple Pear Crisp

Preparation Time: 10 minutes
Cooking Time: 20 minutes
Servings: 4
Ingredients:

- 4 apples, peel, and cut into chunks
- 1 cup steel-cut oats
- 2 pears, cut into chunks
- 1 ½ cup water
- ½ tsp. cinnamon
- ¼ cup maple syrup

Directions:

1. Add all ingredients into the instant pot and stir well.
2. Seal the pot with a lid and cook on manual high for 10 minutes.
3. As soon as done, reduce pressure naturally for 10 minutes and then release it using the quick-release method. Open the lid.
4. Serve warm and enjoy.

Nutrition:

- Calories: 306
- Fat: 1.9 g
- Carbohydrates: 74 g
- Sugar: 45.3 g
- Protein: 3.7 g
- Cholesterol: 0 mg

139.   Vanilla Peanut Butter Fudge

Preparation Time: 10 minutes
Cooking Time: 90 minutes
Servings: 12
Ingredients:

- 1 cup chocolate chips
- 8.5 oz. cream cheese
- ¼ cup peanut butter
- ½ tsp vanilla
- ¼ cup swerve

Directions:

1. Add all ingredients into the instant pot and stir well.
2. Seal the pot with a lid and cook on slow cook mode for 60 minutes.
3. Once done, release pressure using the quick-release method, then open the lid.
4. Stir until smooth and cook for 30 minutes more on sauté mode.
5. Pour mixture into the baking pan and place in the fridge until set.

6. Slice and serve.

Nutrition:

- Calories: 177
- Fat: 13.9 g
- Carbohydrates: 14.9 g
- Sugar: 12.8 g
- Protein: 3.9 g
- Cholesterol: 25 mg

140.   Walnut Carrot Cake

Preparation Time: 10 minutes
Cooking Time: 40 minutes
Servings: 8
Ingredients:

- 3 eggs
- 1 tsp baking powder
- 2/3 cup swerve
- 1 cup almond flour
- ¾ cup walnuts, chopped
- 1 cup carrot, shredded
- ½ cup heavy cream
- ¼ cup coconut oil
- 1 tsp apple pie spice

Directions:

1. Cover a baking dish with cooking spray and set it aside.
2. Add all ingredients into a large bowl and mix with a hand mixer until well combined.
3. Pour batter into the baking dish and cover the dish with foil.
4. Pour 2 cups of water into the instant pot, then place a trivet in the pot.
5. Place the cake dish on top of the trivet.
6. Seal the pot with the lid and cook on manual high pressure for 40 minutes.
7. As soon as done, reduce pressure naturally for 10 minutes and then release it using the quick-release method. Open the lid.
8. Carefully remove the dish from the pot and let it cool.
9. Slice and serve.

Nutrition:

- Calories: 208
- Fat: 19.9 g
- Carbohydrates: 24.1 g
- Sugar: 21.1 g
- Protein: 5.9 g
- Cholesterol: 72 mg

Chapter 9.   Vegetarian Recipes

141.   Fried Peppers with Sriracha Mayo

Preparation Time: 20 minutes
Cooking Time: 10 minutes
Servings: 2
Ingredients:

- 4 bell peppers, seeded and sliced (1-inch pieces)
- 1 onion, sliced (1-inch pieces)
- 1 Tbsp olive oil
- ½ tsp dried rosemary
- ½ tsp dried basil
- Kosher salt, to taste
- ¼ tsp ground black pepper
- 1/3 cup mayonnaise
- 1/3 tsp Sriracha

Directions:

1. Fling the bell peppers and onions with olive oil, rosemary, basil, salt, and black pepper.
2. Place the peppers and onions on an even layer in the cooking basket. Cook at 400°F for 12 to 14 minutes.
3. Meanwhile, make the sauce by whisking the mayonnaise and Sriracha. Serve immediately.

Nutrition:

- Calories: 346
- Fat: 34.1 g
- Carbs: 9.5 g
- Protein: 2.3 g
- Sugars: 4.9 g

142.   Classic Fried Pickles

Preparation Time: 20 minutes
Cooking Time: 10 minutes
Servings: 2
Ingredients:

- 1 egg, whisked
- 2 Tbsp buttermilk
- ½ cup fresh breadcrumbs
- ¼ cup Romano cheese, grated
- ½ tsp onion powder
- ½ tsp garlic powder
- 1 ½ cups dill pickle chips, pressed dry with kitchen towels

Mayo Sauce:

- ¼ cup mayonnaise
- ½ Tbsp mustard
- ½ tsp molasses
- 1 Tbsp ketchup
- ¼ tsp ground black pepper

Directions:

1. In a small bowl, whisk the egg with buttermilk.
2. In another bowl, mix the breadcrumbs, cheese, onion powder, and garlic powder.
3. Dip the pickle chips in the egg mixture, then in the breadcrumb/cheese mixture.
4. Cook in the preheated Air Fryer at 400°F for 5 minutes; shake the basket and cook for 5 minutes more.
5. Meanwhile, mix all the sauce ingredients until well combined. Serve the fried pickles with the mayo sauce for dipping.

Nutrition:

- Calories: 342
- Fat: 28.5 g
- Carbs: 12.5 g
- Protein: 9.1 g
- Sugars: 4.9 g

143.   Fried Green Beans with Pecorino Romano

Preparation Time: 15 minutes
Cooking Time: 10 minutes
Servings: 3
Ingredients:

- 2 Tbsp buttermilk
- 1 egg
- 4 Tbsp cornmeal
- 4 Tbsp tortilla chips, crushed
- 4 Tbsp Pecorino Romano cheese, finely grated
- Coarse salt and crushed black pepper, to taste
- 1 tsp smoked paprika
- 12 oz. green beans, trimmed

Directions:

1. In a small bowl, whisk together the buttermilk and egg.
2. In a separate bowl, combine the cornmeal, tortilla chips, Pecorino Romano cheese, salt, black pepper, and paprika.
3. Dip the green beans in the egg mixture, then in the cornmeal/cheese mixture. Place the green beans in the lightly greased cooking basket.

4. Cook in the preheated Air Fryer at 390°F for 4 minutes. Shake the basket and cook for a further 3 minutes.
5. Taste, adjust the seasonings, and serve with the dipping sauce if desired. Bon appétit!

Nutrition:
- Calories: 340
- Fat: 9.7 g
- Carbs: 50.9 g
- Protein: 12.8 g
- Sugars: 4.7 g

144.   Spicy Glazed Carrots

Preparation Time: 20 minutes
Cooking Time: 10 minutes
Servings: 3

Ingredients:
- 1 lb. carrots, cut into matchsticks
- 2 Tbsp peanut oil
- 1 Tbsp agave syrup
- 1 jalapeño, seeded and minced
- ¼ tsp dill
- ½ tsp basil
- Salt and white pepper, to taste

Directions:
1. Jolt by warming your Air Fryer to 380°F.
2. Toss all ingredients together and place them in the Air Fryer basket.
3. Cook for 15 minutes, shaking the basket halfway through the cooking time. Transfer to a serving platter and enjoy!

Nutrition:
- Calories: 162
- Fat: 9.3 g
- Carbs: 20.1 g
- Protein: 1.4 g
- Sugars: 12.8 g

145.   Corn on the Cob with Herb Butter

Preparation Time: 15 minutes
Cooking Time: 10 minutes
Servings: 2

Ingredients:
- 2 ears new corn, shucked and cut into halves
- 2 Tbsp butter, room temperature
- 1 tsp granulated garlic
- ½ tsp fresh ginger, grated
- Sea salt and pepper, to taste
- 1 Tbsp fresh rosemary, chopped
- 1 Tbsp fresh basil, chopped
- 2 Tbsp fresh chives, roughly chopped

Directions:
1. Cover the corn with cooking spray. Cook at 395°F for 6 minutes, turning them over halfway through the cooking time.
2. For the time being, mix the butter with the granulated garlic, ginger, salt, black pepper, rosemary, and basil.
3. Spread the butter mixture all over the corn on the cob. Cook in the preheated Air Fryer for an additional 2 minutes. Bon appétit!

Nutrition:
- Calories: 239
- Fat: 13.3 g
- Carbs: 30.2 g
- Protein: 5.4 g
- Sugars: 5.8 g

146.   Rainbow Vegetable Fritters

Preparation Time: 20 minutes
Cooking Time: 10 minutes
Servings: 2

Ingredients:
- 1 zucchini, grated and squeezed
- 1 cup corn kernels
- ½ cup canned green peas
- 4 Tbsp all-purpose flour
- 2 Tbsp fresh shallots, minced
- 1 tsp fresh garlic, minced
- 1 Tbsp peanut oil
- Sea salt and pepper, to taste
- 1 tsp cayenne pepper

Directions:
1. In a mixing bowl, thoroughly combine all ingredients until everything is well incorporated.
2. Shape the mixture into patties. Cover the Air Fryer carrier with cooking spray.
3. Cook in the preheated Air Fryer at 365°F for 6 minutes. Flip them over and cook for a further 6 minutes
4. Serve immediately and enjoy!

Nutrition:
- Calories: 215
- Fat: 8.4 g
- Carbs: 31.6 g
- Protein: 6 g
- Sugars: 4.1 g

147. Mediterranean Vegetable Skewers

Preparation Time: 30 minutes
Cooking Time: 10 minutes
Servings: 4
Ingredients:

- 2 medium-sized zucchinis, cut into 1-inch pieces
- 2 red bell peppers, cut into 1-inch pieces
- 1 green bell pepper, cut into 1-inch pieces
- 1 red onion, cut into 1-inch pieces
- 2 Tbsp olive oil
- Sea salt, to taste
- ½ tsp black pepper, preferably freshly cracked
- ½ tsp red pepper flakes

Directions:

1. Soak the wooden skewers in water for 15 minutes.
2. Thread the vegetables on skewers, drizzle olive oil all over the vegetable skewers, sprinkle with spices.
3. Cook in the preheated Air Fryer at 400°F for 13 minutes. Serve warm and enjoy!

Nutrition:

- Calories: 138
- Fat: 10.2 g
- Carbs: 10.2 g
- Protein: 2.2 g
- Sugars: 6.6 g

148. Roasted Veggies with Yogurt-Tahini Sauce

Preparation Time: 20 minutes
Cooking Time: 10 minutes
Servings: 4
Ingredients:

- 1 lb. Brussels sprouts
- 1 lb. button mushrooms
- 2 Tbsp olive oil
- ½ tsp white pepper
- ½ tsp dried dill weed
- ½ tsp cayenne pepper
- ½ tsp celery seeds
- ½ tsp mustard seeds
- Salt, to taste

Yogurt Tahini Sauce:

- 1 cup plain yogurt
- 2 heaping Tbsp tahini paste
- 1 Tbsp lemon juice
- 1 Tbsp extra-virgin olive oil
- ½ tsp Aleppo pepper, minced

Directions:

1. Toss the Brussels sprouts and mushrooms with olive oil and spices. Preheat your Air Fryer to 380°F.
2. Add the Brussels sprouts to the cooking basket and cook for 10 minutes.
3. Add the mushrooms, turn the temperature to 390°F and cook for 6 minutes more.
4. While the vegetables are cooking, make the sauce by whisking all ingredients. Serve the warm vegetables with the sauce on the side. Bon appétit!

Nutrition:

- Calories: 254
- Fat: 17.2 g
- Carbs: 19.6 g
- Protein: 11.1 g
- Sugars: 8.1 g

149. Swiss Cheese and Vegetable Casserole

Preparation Time: 50 minutes
Cooking Time: 10 minutes
Servings: 4
Ingredients:

- 1 lb. potatoes, peeled and sliced (1/4-inch thick
- 2 Tbsp olive oil
- ½ tsp red pepper flakes, crushed
- ½ tsp freshly ground black pepper
- Salt, to taste
- 3 bell peppers, thinly sliced
- 1 serrano pepper, thinly sliced
- 2 medium-sized tomatoes, sliced
- 1 leek, thinly sliced
- 2 garlic cloves, minced
- 1 cup Swiss cheese, shredded

Directions:

1. Start by warming your Air Fryer to 350°F. Cover a casserole dish with cooking oil.
2. Place the potatoes in the casserole dish in an even layer; drizzle 1 Tbsp of olive oil over the top, then swell the red pepper, black pepper, and salt.
3. Add 2 bell peppers and 1/2 of the leeks. Add the tomatoes and the remaining 1 Tbsp of olive oil.
4. Add the remaining peppers, leeks, and minced garlic. Top with the cheese.
5. Cover the casserole with foil and bake for 32 minutes. Remove the foil and increase the temperature to 400°F; bake an additional 16 minutes. Bon appétit!

Nutrition:

- Calories: 328
- Fat: 16.5 g

- Carbs: 33.1 g
- Protein: 13.1 g
- Sugars: 7.6 g

150. American-Style Brussels Sprout Salad

Preparation Time: 35 minutes
Cooking Time: 10 minutes
Servings: 4
Ingredients:

- 1 lb. Brussels sprouts
- 1 apple, cored and diced
- ½ cup mozzarella cheese, crumbled
- ½ cup pomegranate seeds
- 1 small-sized red onion, chopped
- 4 eggs, hardboiled and sliced

Dressing:

- ¼ cup olive oil
- 2 Tbsp champagne vinegar
- 1 tsp Dijon mustard
- 1 tsp honey
- Sea salt and ground black pepper, to taste

Directions:

1. Start by preheating your Air Fryer to 380°F.
2. Add the Brussels sprouts to the cooking basket. Cover with cooking spray and cook for 15 minutes. Let it cool to room temperature for about 15 minutes.
3. Toss the Brussels sprouts with the apple, cheese, pomegranate seeds, and red onion.
4. Mix all ingredients for the dressing and toss to combine well. Serve topped with hard-boiled eggs. Bon appétit!

Nutrition:

- Calories: 319
- Fat: 18.5 g
- Carbs: 27 g
- Protein: 14.7 g
- Sugars: 14.6 g

151. The Best Cauliflower Tater Tots

Preparation Time: 25 minutes
Cooking Time: 10 minutes
Servings: 4
Ingredients:

- 1 lb. cauliflower florets
- 2 eggs
- 1 Tbsp olive oil
- 2 Tbsp scallions, chopped
- 1 garlic clove, minced
- 1 cup Colby cheese, shredded

- ½ cup breadcrumbs
- Sea salt and ground black pepper, to taste
- ¼ tsp dried dill weed
- 1 tsp paprika

Directions:

1. Blanch the cauliflower in salted boiling water for about 3 to 4 minutes until al dente. Drain well and pulse in a food processor.
2. Add the remaining ingredients; mix to combine well. Shape the cauliflower mixture into bite-sized tots.
3. Cover the Air Fryer basket with cooking spray.
4. Cook in the preheated Air Fryer at 375°F for 16 minutes, shaking halfway through the cooking time. Serve with your favorite sauce for dipping. Bon appétit!

Nutrition:

- Calories: 267
- Fat: 19.2 g
- Carbs: 9.6 g
- Protein: 14.9 g
- Sugars: 2.9 g

152. Three-Cheese Stuffed Mushrooms

Preparation Time: 15 minutes
Cooking Time: 10 minutes
Servings: 3
Ingredients:

- 9 large button mushrooms, stems removed
- 1 Tbsp olive oil
- Salt and ground black pepper, to taste
- ½ tsp dried rosemary
- 6 Tbsp Swiss cheese shredded
- 6 Tbsp Romano cheese, shredded
- 6 Tbsp cream cheese
- 1 tsp soy sauce
- 1 tsp garlic, minced
- 3 Tbsp green onion, minced

Directions:

1. Brush the mushroom caps with olive oil; sprinkle with salt, pepper, and rosemary.
2. In a mixing bowl, thoroughly combine the remaining ingredients, mix them well, and divide the filling mixture among the mushroom caps.
3. Cook in the preheated Air Fryer at 390°F for 7 minutes.
4. Let the mushrooms cool slightly before serving. Bon appétit!

Nutrition:

- Calories: 345
- Fat: 28 g

- Carbs: 11.2 g
- Protein: 14.4 g
- Sugars: 8.1 g

153.   Sweet Corn Fritters with Avocado

Preparation Time: 20 minutes
Cooking Time: 10 minutes
Servings: 3
Ingredients:

- 2 cups sweet corn kernels
- 1 small-sized onion, chopped
- 1 garlic clove, minced
- 2 eggs, whisked
- 1 tsp baking powder
- 2 Tbsp fresh cilantro, chopped
- Sea salt and ground black pepper, to taste
- 1 avocado, peeled, pitted, and diced
- 2 Tbsp sweet chili sauce

Directions:

1. In a mixing bowl, thoroughly combine the corn, onion, garlic, eggs, baking powder, cilantro, salt, and black pepper.
2. Shape the corn mixture into 6 patties and transfer them to the lightly greased Air Fryer basket.
3. Cook in the preheated Air Fry at 370°F for 8 minutes; turn them over and cook for 7 minutes longer.
4. Serve the patties with avocado and chili sauce.

Nutrition:

- Calories: 383
- Fat: 21.3 g
- Carbs: 42.8 g
- Protein: 12.7 g
- Sugars: 9.2 g

154.   Greek-Style Vegetable Bake

Preparation Time: 35 minutes
Cooking Time: 10 minutes
Servings: 4
Ingredients:

- 1 eggplant, peeled and sliced
- 2 bell peppers, seeded and sliced
- 1 red onion, sliced
- 1 tsp fresh garlic, minced
- 4 Tbsp olive oil
- 1 tsp mustard
- 1 tsp dried oregano
- 1 tsp smoked paprika
- Salt and ground black pepper, to taste

- 1 tomato, sliced
- 6 oz. halloumi cheese, sliced lengthways

Directions:

1. Start by preheating your Air Fryer to 370°F. Cover a baking pan with nonstick cooking spray.
2. Place the eggplant, peppers, onion, and garlic on the baking pan's bottom. Add the olive oil, mustard, and spices. Transfer to the cooking basket and cook for 14 minutes.
3. Top with the tomatoes and cheese; increase the temperature to 390°F and cook for 5 minutes more until bubbling. Let it sit on a cooling rack for 10 minutes before serving.
4. Bon appétit!

Nutrition:

- Calories: 296
- Fat: 22.9 g
- Carbs: 16.1 g
- Protein: 9.3 g
- Sugars: 9.9 g

155.   Japanese Tempura Bowl

Preparation Time: 20 minutes
Cooking Time: 10 minutes
Servings: 3
Ingredients:

- 1 cup all-purpose flour
- Kosher salt and ground black pepper, to taste
- ½ tsp paprika
- 2 eggs
- 3 Tbsp soda water
- 1 cup panko crumbs
- 2 Tbsp olive oil
- 1 cup green beans
- 1 onion, cut into rings
- 1 zucchini, cut into slices
- 2 Tbsp soy sauce
- 1 Tbsp mirin
- 1 tsp dashi granules

Directions:

1. In a small bowl, mix the flour, salt, black pepper, and paprika. In a separate bowl, whisk the eggs and soda water. In a third shallow bowl, combine the panko crumbs with olive oil.
2. Dip the vegetables in the flour mixture, then in the egg mixture; lastly, roll over the panko mixture to coat evenly.
3. Cook in the preheated Air Fryer at 400°F for 10 minutes, shaking the basket halfway through the cooking time. Work in batches until the vegetables are crispy and golden brown.

4. Then, make the sauce by whisking the soy sauce, mirin and dashi granules. Bon appétit!

Nutrition:
- Calories: 446
- Fat: 14.7 g
- Carbs: 63.5 g
- Protein: 14.6 g
- Sugars: 3.8 g

156.   Balsamic Root Vegetables

Preparation Time: 25 minutes
Cooking Time: 10 minutes
Servings: 3
Ingredients:
- 2 potatoes, cut into 1 1/2-inch piece
- 2 carrots, cut into 1 1/2-inch piece
- 2 parsnips, cut into 1 1/2-inch piece
- 1 onion, cut into 1 1/2-inch piece
- Pink Himalayan salt and ground black pepper, to taste
- ¼ tsp smoked paprika
- 1 tsp garlic powder
- 1/2 tsp dried thyme
- 1/2 tsp dried marjoram
- 2 Tbsp olive oil
- 2 Tbsp balsamic vinegar

Directions:
1. Toss all ingredients in a large mixing dish.
2. Roast in the preheated Air Fryer at 400°F for 10 minutes. Shake the basket and cook for 7 minutes more.
3. Serve with some extra fresh herbs if desired. Bon appétit!

Nutrition:
- Calories: 405
- Fat: 9.7 g
- Carbs: 74.7 g
- Protein: 7.7 g
- Sugars: 15.2 g

157.   Winter Vegetable Braise

Preparation Time: 25 minutes
Cooking Time: 10 minutes
Servings: 2
Ingredients:
- 4 potatoes, peeled and cut into 1-inch pieces
- 1 celery root, peeled and cut into 1-inch pieces
- 1 cup winter squash
- 2 Tbsp unsalted butter, melted

- ½ cup chicken broth
- ¼ cup tomato sauce
- 1 tsp parsley
- 1 tsp rosemary
- 1 tsp thyme

Directions:
1. Start by preheating your Air Fryer to 370°F. Add all ingredients to a lightly greased casserole dish. Stir to combine well.
2. Bake in the preheated Air Fryer for 10 minutes. Gently stir the vegetables with a large spoon and increase the temperature to 400°F; cook for 10 minutes more.
3. Serve in individual bowls with a few drizzles of lemon juice. Bon appétit!

Nutrition:
- Calories: 358
- Fat: 12.3 g
- Carbs: 55.7 g
- Protein: 7.7 g
- Sugars: 7.4 g

158.   Family Vegetable Gratin

Preparation Time: 35 minutes
Cooking Time: 10 minutes
Servings: 4
Ingredients:
- 1 lb. Chinese cabbage, roughly chopped
- 2 bell peppers, seeded and sliced
- 1 jalapeno pepper, seeded and sliced
- 1 onion, thickly sliced
- 2 garlic cloves, sliced
- 1/2 stick butter
- 4 Tbsp all-purpose flour
- 1 cup milk
- 1 cup cream cheese
- Sea salt and freshly ground black pepper, to taste
- 1/2 tsp cayenne pepper
- 1 cup Monterey Jack cheese, shredded

Directions:
1. Heat a pan with salted water and bring to a boil. Boil the Chinese cabbage for 2 to 3 minutes. Transfer the Chinese cabbage to cold water to stop the cooking process.
2. Place the Chinese cabbage in a lightly greased casserole dish. Add the peppers, onion, and garlic.
3. Next, melt the butter in a saucepan over moderate heat. Gradually add the flour and cook for 2 minutes to form a paste.
4. Slowly pour in the milk, stirring continuously until a thick sauce forms. Add the cream cheese.

5. Season with salt, black pepper, and cayenne pepper. Add the mixture to the casserole dish.
6. Top with the shredded Monterey Jack cheese and bake in the preheated Air Fryer at 390°F for 25 minutes. Serve hot.

Nutrition:
- Calories: 373
- Fat: 26.1 g
- Carbs: 17.7 g
- Protein: 18.7 g
- Sugars. 7.7 g

159.   Sweet-and-Sour Mixed Veggies

Preparation Time: 25 minutes
Cooking Time: 10 minutes
Servings: 4
Ingredients:
- ½ lb. sterling asparagus, cut into 1 1/2-inch piece
- ½ lb. broccoli, cut into 1 1/2-inch piece
- ½ lb. carrots, cut into 1 1/2-inch piece
- 2 Tbsp peanut oil
- Some salt and white pepper, to taste
- ½ cup water
- 4 Tbsp raisins
- 2 Tbsp honey
- 2 Tbsp apple cider vinegar

Directions:
1. Place the vegetables in a single layer in the lightly greased cooking basket. Drizzle the peanut oil over the vegetables.
2. Sprinkle with salt and white pepper.
3. Cook at 380°F for 15 minutes, shaking the basket halfway through the cooking time.
4. Add 1/2 cup of water to a saucepan; bring to a rapid boil and add the raisins, honey, and vinegar. Prepare for 5 to 7 minutes or until the sauce has been reduced by half.
5. Spoon the sauce over the warm vegetables and serve immediately. Bon appétit!

Nutrition:
- Calories: 153
- Fat: 7.1 g
- Carbs: 21.6 g
- Protein: 3.6 g
- Sugars: 14.2 g

160.   Carrot and Oat Balls

Preparation Time: 25 minutes
Cooking Time: 10 minutes
Servings: 3
Ingredients:
- 4 carrots, grated
- 1 cup rolled oats, ground
- 1 Tbsp butter, room temperature
- 1 Tbsp chia seeds
- ½ cup scallions, chopped
- 2 cloves garlic, minced
- 2 Tbsp tomato ketchup
- 1 tsp cayenne pepper
- ½ tsp sea salt
- ¼ tsp ground black pepper
- ½ tsp ancho chili powder
- ¼ cup fresh bread crumbs

Directions:
1. Start by preheating your Air Fryer to 380°F.
2. In a bowl, mix all ingredients until everything is well incorporated. Shape the batter into bite-sized balls.
3. Cook the balls for 15 minutes, shaking the basket halfway through the cooking time. Bon appétit!

Nutrition:
- Calories: 215
- Fat: 4.7 g
- Carbs. 37.2 g
- Protein: 7.5 g
- Sugars: 5.6 g

Chapter 10.   30 Day Meal Plan

Day	Breakfast	Lunch	Dinner
1	Air Fryer Hard Boiled Eggs	Beef Korma Curry	Mustard-Crusted Sole
2	Air Fryer Grilled Cheese Sandwiches	Chicken Fried Steak	Almond Crusted Cod with Chips
3	Air Fryer Hot Dogs	Lemon Greek Beef and Vegetables	Honey Lemon Snapper with Fruit
4	Air Fryer Perfect Cinnamon Toast	Country-Style Pork Ribs	Easy Tuna Wraps
5	Air Fryer Monkey Bread	Lemon and Honey Pork Tenderloin	Asian-Inspired Swordfish Steaks
6	Air Fryer Bacon	Dijon Pork Tenderloin	Salmon with Fennel and Carrot
7	Air Fryer Meatballs in Tomato Sauce	Air Fryer Pork Satay	Ranch Tilapia fillets
8	Chicken Fried Spring Rolls	Pork Burgers with Red Cabbage Slaw	Chilean Sea Bass with Green Olive Relish
9	Mushroom and Cheese Frittata	Greek Lamb Pita Pockets	Ginger and Green Onion Fish
10	Cinnamon and Cheese Pancake	Rosemary Lamb Chops	Asian Sesame Cod
11	Low-Carb White Egg and Spinach Frittata	Delicious Meatballs	Lemon Scallops with Asparagus
12	Scallion Sandwich	Low-fat Steak	Fish Tacos
13	Lean Lamb and Turkey Meatballs with Yogurt	Diet Boiled Ribs	Spicy Cajun Shrimp
14	Air Fried Eggs	Meatloaf	Garlic Parmesan Roasted Shrimp
15	Cinnamon Pancake	Beef with Mushrooms	Quick Shrimp Scampi
16	Spinach and Mushrooms Omelet	Warm Chicken and Spinach Salad	Fried Peppers with Sriracha Mayo
17	All Berries Pancakes	Chicken in Tomato Juice	Classic Fried Pickles
18	Cinnamon Overnight Oats	Chicken Wings with Curry	Fried Green Beans with Pecorino Romano
19	Ham and Cheese English Muffin Melt	Chicken Meatballs	Spicy Glazed Carrots
20	Asparagus Omelet	Stuffed Chicken	Corn on the Cob with Herb Butter
21	Pumpkin Pie French Toast	Duo Crisp Chicken Wings	Rainbow Vegetable Fritters
22	Breakfast Cheese Bread Cups	Italian Whole Chicken	Mediterranean Vegetable Skewers
23	Breakfast Cod Nuggets	Chicken Pot Pie	Roasted Veggies with Yogurt-Tahini Sauce
24	Vegetable Egg Pancake	Chicken Casserole	Swiss Cheese and Vegetable Casserole
25	Oriental Omelet	Ranch Chicken Wings	American-Style Brussels Sprout Salad

26	Crispy Breakfast Avocado Fries	Chicken Mac and Cheese	The Best Cauliflower Tater Tots
27	Cheese and Egg Breakfast Sandwich	Broccoli Chicken Casserole	Three-Cheese Stuffed Mushrooms
28	Baked Mini Quiche	Chicken Tikka Kebab	Sweet Corn Fritters with Avocado
29	Peanut Butter and Banana Breakfast Sandwich	Bacon-Wrapped Chicken	Greek-Style Vegetable Bake
30	Eggs and Cocotte on Toast	Creamy Chicken Thighs	Japanese Tempura Bowl

Chapter 11. Conclusion

Diabetic Air-Fryer Cookbook cookware is ideal for diabetic air-fryers as it cooks evenly and quickly so you can enjoy more time to talk and eat with your loved ones. You will be able to stir-fry food and toast bread with Diabetic Air-Fryer Cookbook cookware, all without sacrificing quality or cleanliness. In addition to being durable, Diabetic Air-Fryer Cookbook cookware is nonstick, so you won't have to waste your time spending ages scrubbing your pans after each use. With a reversible stainless-steel handle, you can carry your air fryer in your hands or on your hip for easy one-hand operation.

Worth buying? Yes! Suppose you're looking for an air fryer that cooks food more healthily. In that case, you need to look at a Diabetic Air-Fryer Cookbook air fryer and other products from the Diabetic Air-Fryer Cookbook Company. Diabetic Air-Fryer Cookbook Air Fryers are a great way to cook healthy foods, but it's important to recognize that cooking can be dangerous if you don't know what you're doing. Cooking safely is essential for anyone who is diabetic or tight on time. To make sure your air fryer stays safe, we wrote Diabetic Air Fryer Cookbook to help you learn how to cook safely.

At Diabetic Air-Fryer Cookbook, we understand that our products' quality is just as important as the quality of our service. That is why we stand behind them with a 12-month warranty. Our warranty covers manufacturing defects and defects in materials and quality.

Take the worry out of your diet with this cookbook brought to you by Diabetic Air-Fryer Cookbook. It contains all the recipes you need to make healthy meals for your family. Included are easy-to-follow instructions for preparing healthy meals during a fast or when you have diabetes. You'll also find ideas for using other foods on your Nutrisystem shopping lists like fresh fruits and vegetables.

The Diabetic Air-Fryer Cookbook is a set of recipes designed for people with diabetes who also have hypoglycemia or low blood sugar. The recipes serve as a quick way to reduce your blood sugar level after eating foods that might cause a hypoglycemic reaction. These recipes were created by registered dieticians and diabetes experts who offer fast and simple options that people with diabetes can enjoy.

This cookbook offers solutions for common situations in which your blood glucose level might go too high, too low, or stay too high for too long after you eat. It covers sweet treats, which might cause more rapid reactions than savory dishes. This cookbook offers over 100 recipes related to these situations, including salt and vinegar potato chips, chocolate-covered cherries, dried apricots, banana oatmeal muffins, and more.

This cookbook is dedicated to anyone who has a family member with diabetes. We know how hard it can be to prepare delicious meals, especially in times of stress and busy schedules! That's why we have written this cookbook. We hope our recipes will help you get back to the good cooking you used to do. We want you to be happy with what you prepare and how you feel when you eat it.

If your family member has diabetes, we are sure they will appreciate your advance notice, careful attention, and the thoughtfulness behind the ingredients that go into each recipe. Hopefully, you will find something in this book that your diabetic family member will like or want to try.

Sometimes cooking for someone with diabetes is difficult. You are probably already aware of this — hoping that the instructions in this book are followed precisely so it will help give everyone involved confidence in what they have prepared. This is a good thing — there are some significant results when faithfulness is given regarding every recipe.

Some tips may help prepare fresh foods and dishes for a diabetic person. With a little planning, everyone can be happy with any meal or snack results they prepare.